Trace Minerals in Ruminants

Editors

WILLIAM S. SWECKER JR
ROBERT J. VAN SAUN

VETERINARY CLINICS OF NORTH AMERICA: FOOD ANIMAL PRACTICE

www.vetfood.theclinics.com

Consulting Editor
ROBERT A. SMITH

November 2023 • Volume 39 • Number 3

ELSEVIER

1600 John F. Kennedy Boulevard ● Suite 1800 ● Philadelphia, Pennsylvania, 19103-2899

http://www.vetfood.theclinics.com

**VETERINARY CLINICS OF NORTH AMERICA: FOOD ANIMAL PRACTICE Volume 39, Number 3
November 2023 ISSN 0749-0720, ISBN-13: 978-0-443-18342-3**

Editor: Taylor Hayes
Developmental Editor: Varun Gopal

Veterinary Clinics of North America: Food Animal Practice (ISSN 0749-0720) is published in March, July, and November by Elsevier Inc., 360 Park Avenue South, New York, NY 10010-1710. Subscription prices are $267.00 per year (domestic individuals), $533.00 per year (domestic institutions), $100.00 per year (domestic students/residents), $289.00 per year (Canadian individuals), $702.00 per year (Canadian institutions), $342.00 per year (international individuals), $702.00 per year (international institutions), $100.00 per year (Canadian students), and $165.00 (international students). To receive student/resident rate, orders must be accompanied by name of affiliated institution, date of term, and the signature of program/residency coordinator on institution letterhead. *Clinics* subscription prices. All prices are subject to change without notice. **POSTMASTER:** Send address changes to *Veterinary Clinics of North America: Food Animal Practice*, Elsevier Health Sciences Division, Subscription Customer Service, 3251 Riverport Lane, Maryland Heights, MO 63043. Customer Service (orders, claims, online, change of address): Elsevier Health Sciences Division, Subscription **Customer Service, 3251 Riverport Lane, Maryland Heights, MO 63043. Tel: 1-800-654-2452 (U.S. and Canada); 314-447-8871 (ouside U.S. and Canada). Fax: 314-447-8029. E-mail: journalscustomerservice-usa@elsevier.com (for print support); journalsonlinesupport-usa@elsevier.com (for online support).**

Reprints. For copies of 100 or more, of articles in this publication, please contact the Commercial Reprints Department, Elsevier Inc., 360 Park Avenue South, New York, NY 10010-1710. Tel.: 212-633-3874; Fax: 212-633-3820; E-mail: reprints@elsevier.com.

Veterinary Clinics of North America: Food Animal Practice is covered in *Current Contents/Agriculture, Biology and Environmental Sciences, MEDLINE/PubMed (Index Medicus), and Excerpta Medica.*

Contributors

CONSULTING EDITOR

ROBERT A. SMITH, DVM, MS
Diplomate, American Board of Veterinary Practitioners; Veterinary Research and Consulting Services, LLC, Greeley, Colorado; Veterinary Research and Consulting Services, LLC, Stillwater, Oklahoma, USA

EDITORS

WILLIAM S. SWECKER Jr, DVM, PhD
Diplomate, American College of Veterinary Internal Medicine (Nutrition); Professor and Director, Veterinary Teaching Hospital, Virginia-Maryland Regional College of Veterinary Medicine, Virginia Tech, Blacksburg, Virginia, USA

ROBERT J. VAN SAUN, DVM, MS, PhD
Diplomate, American College of Theriogenologists; Diplomate, American College of Veterinary Internal Medicine (Nutrition); Professor of Veterinary Science and Extension Veterinarian, Department of Veterinary and Biomedical Sciences, College of Agricultural Sciences, Pennsylvania State University, University Park, Pennsylvania, USA

AUTHORS

PAUL A. BECK, MS, PhD, MBA
State Extension Beef Cattle Nutrition Specialist, Department of Animal and Food Sciences, Oklahoma State University, Stillwater, Oklahoma, USA

JOHN P. BUCHWEITZ, PhD
Diplomate, American Board of Toxicology; Associate Professor, Department of Pathobiology and Diagnostic Investigation, College of Veterinary Medicine, Michigan State University, East Lansing, Michigan, USA; MSU Veterinary Diagnostic Laboratory, Lansing, Michigan, USA

ROBERT B. CORBETT, DVM, PAS
Diplomate, American College of Animal Nutrition; President, Dairy Health Consultation, Spring City, Utah, USA

LILY N. EDWARDS-CALLAWAY, PhD
Department of Animal Science, Colorado State University, Fort Collins, Colorado, USA

TERRY E. ENGLE, PhD, PAS
Department of Animal Science, Professor and Associate Department Head Animal Sciences, Colorado State University, Fort Collins, Colorado, USA

HELEN M. GOLDER, BAgSc (Hons), PhD
Scibus, Dairy Science Group, School of Life and Environmental Sciences, Faculty of Science, The University of Sydney, Camden, New South Wales, Australia

JEFFERY O. HALL, DVM, PhD
Diplomate, American Board of Veterinary Toxicology; Cattle Technical Services Veterinarian, Huvepharma Inc, Wellsville, Utah, USA

IAN J. LEAN, BVSc, DVSc, PhD, MANZCVS
Scibus, Dairy Science Group, School of Life and Environmental Sciences, Faculty of Science, The University of Sydney, Camden, New South Wales, Australia

DAVID G. PUGH, DVM, MS, MAG
Diplomate, American College of Theriogenology; Diplomate, American College of Veterinary Internal Medicine (Nutrition); Diplomate, American College of Veterinary Microbiology (Parasitology); SouthernTraxx Veterinary Services, Waverly, Alabama, USA

BIRGIT PUSCHNER, DVM, PhD
Diplomate, American Board of Veterinary Toxicology; Professor, Department of Pathobiology and Diagnostic Investigation, College of Veterinary Medicine, Michigan State University, East Lansing, Michigan, USA; MSU Veterinary Diagnostic Laboratory, Lansing, Michigan, USA

BOB SAGER, DVM, PhD
Diplomate, American Board of Veterinary Practitioners (Beef Cattle Practice); Medicine Creek Bovine Health and Consulting, White Sulphur Springs, Montana, USA

RACHEL SHEFFLER, DVM
Department of Pathobiology and Diagnostic Investigation, College of Veterinary Medicine, Michigan State University, East Lansing, Michigan, USA; MSU Veterinary Diagnostic Laboratory, Lansing, Michigan, USA

JERRY W. SPEARS, PhD
Professor Emeritus, Department of Animal Science, North Carolina State University, Raleigh, North Carolina, USA

WILLIAM S. SWECKER Jr, DVM, PhD
Diplomate, American College of Veterinary Internal Medicine (Nutrition); Professor and Director, Veterinary Teaching Hospital, Virginia-Maryland Regional College of Veterinary Medicine, Virginia Tech, Blacksburg, Virginia, USA

ROBERT J. VAN SAUN, DVM, MS, PhD
Diplomate, American College of Theriogenologists; Diplomate, American College of Veterinary Internal Medicine (Nutrition); Professor of Veterinary Science and Extension Veterinarian, Department of Veterinary and Biomedical Sciences, College of Agricultural Sciences, Pennsylvania State University, University Park, Pennsylvania, USA

JOHN J. WAGNER, PhD, PAS
Department of Animal Science, Colorado State University, Fort Collins, Colorado, USA

Contents

Trace minerals are commonly supplemented in ruminant feeds as many common feeds are deficient in one or more of the trace minerals. The requirement of trace minerals needed to prevent classic nutrient deficiencies is well established, thus those cases most commonly occur when no supplement is provided. The more common challenge for the practitioner is to determine if additional supplementation is needed to enhance production or decrease disease occurrence.

Trace minerals are essential nutrients that have many biologic functions, many of which are related to metabolic activities, immune function, and antioxidant capacity. The pregnant dam provides essential nutrients to support fetal development, including trace minerals. Milk is known to be an insufficient source of many trace minerals during the early nursing neonatal period. The fetal liver is capable of concentrating minerals to generate a reserve for use during postnatal life; however, the sufficiency of this reserve is dependent upon maternal mineral status. Appropriate mineral supplementation in the gestational diet is critical to supporting fetal development, maintaining adequate antioxidant capacity to survive the birthing process, and sustain immune function and growth of the newborn animal.

Several trace mineral sources, including inorganic, numerous organic, and hydroxychloride sources, are available for dietary supplementation or inclusion in a free-choice supplement. Inorganic forms of copper and manganese differ in their bioavailability. Although research results have been variable, organic and hydroxychloride trace minerals are generally considered more bioavailable than inorganic sources. Research indicates that fiber digestibility is lower in ruminants fed sulfate trace minerals compared with hydroxychloride and some organic sources. Compared with free-choice supplements, individual dosing with rumen boluses or injectable forms ensures that each animal receives the same quantity of a trace mineral.

Veterinarians are often called upon to diagnose health-related issues on the farm that may be related to trace mineral deficiencies or toxicities. Trace mineral feeding rates are often not available due to the proprietary nature of the trace mineral premixes provided by nutritional consultants. The veterinarian needs to be aware of the common clinical signs of trace mineral deficiencies and toxicities, interactions between trace minerals that may result in deficiencies, clinical samples that are necessary for the proper diagnosis, and the recommended normal ranges of each trace mineral depending on the age of the animal.

 Video content accompanies this article at http://www.vetfood. theclinics.com.

While mineral requirements do not differ with the production systems, the forage bases of the different dairy production systems influence the risk of mineral deficiency. Testing representative pastures on a farm is a key to understanding the potential for risk of mineral deficiency and should be combined with blood or tissue samples, clinical observation, and responses to treatment to evaluate the need for supplementation.

The United States Department of Agriculture defines pastureland as "A land cover/use category of land managed primarily for the production of introduced forage plants for livestock grazing." The purpose of this article is to review trace mineral supplementation for beef cattle in this environment. Supplementation of trace minerals in these environments is accomplished with the use of a trace mineralized salt or a complete mineral-vitamin product that contains macrominerals, trace minerals, and vitamins. The form of the supplement may influence uptake and utilization. Supplementation may be augmented with pulse dosing with injectables or oral products.

Range mineral supplementation is based on providing trace minerals not adequately provided from grazed forage in meeting beef cattle needs throughout life cycle stages. Supplementation programs should be developed with consideration of ranch production goals, economics, and practicality for implementation. Factors such as season of grazing, forage analysis, water analysis including antagonistic elements, and measured animal responses are used in mineral supplement formulation for range cattle. Mineral intake is a critical factor to a supplement program's success. Salt-based mineral products are most used under range conditions, yet there is much individual intake variation.

This article reviews the trace mineral and macro mineral content of small grain forages and the potential role in the health of cattle grazing the forages. Reasons for the variability of trace mineral content in small grain forages are discussed, as well as the role of antagonists, such as sulfur and molybdenum, in creating trace mineral deficiencies. The sampling of cattle for the determination of trace mineral statues is described, including which samples to collect for analysis, as well as sample handling. The authors offer a useful discussion on the vitamin content of small grain forages, and conclude that vitamin supplementation is not necessary.

Trace minerals and vitamins are essential for optimizing feedlot cattle growth, health, and carcass characteristics. Understanding factors that influence trace mineral and vitamin absorption and metabolism is important when formulating feedlot cattle diets. Current feedlot industry supplementation practices typically exceed published trace mineral requirements by a factor of 2 to 4. Therefore, the intent of this review is to briefly discuss the functions of trace minerals and vitamins that are typically supplemented in feedlot diets and to examine the impact of dose of trace mineral or vitamin on growth performance, health, and carcass characteristics of feedlot cattle.

Trace mineral nutrition of sheep often focuses on their greater susceptibility to copper toxicosis due to a lesser biliary excretion ability compared with other ruminants. Our understanding of sheep trace mineral requirements has improved for most elements allowing for a factorial approach to determining daily requirement instead of a dietary concentration. Forage trace mineral content is influenced by many factors making issues of trace mineral supplementation geographic-dependent. Oral delivery of trace elements is a preferred supplementation method, and this can be achieved through free choice trace mineralized salt or direct dietary incorporation.

This article is an overview of trace mineral nutrition, disease association with dietary inadequacy of trace minerals, and the associated diseases in goats. The trace minerals most commonly associated with deficiency-related diseases encountered in clinical veterinary medicine, Copper, Zinc, and Selenium, are discussed in greater detail than those less commonly associated with diseases. However, Cobalt, Iron, and Iodine are also discussed. The signs of deficiency-associated diseases, along with diagnostic evaluation to confirm such diseases, are also discussed.

> Veterinarians are often called upon to diagnose health-related issues on the farm that may be related to trace mineral deficiencies or toxicities. Trace mineral feeding rates are often not available due to the proprietary nature of the trace mineral premixes provided by nutritional consultants. The veterinarian needs to be aware of the common clinical signs of trace mineral deficiencies and toxicities, interactions between trace minerals that may result in deficiencies, clinical samples that are necessary for the proper diagnosis, and the recommended normal ranges of each trace mineral depending on the age of the animal.

VETERINARY CLINICS OF NORTH AMERICA: FOOD ANIMAL PRACTICE

THE CLINICS ARE NOW AVAILABLE ONLINE!
Access your subscription at:
www.theclinics.com

Preface

Trace Minerals in Ruminant Production Systems

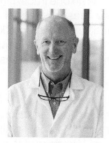   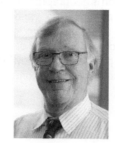

William S. Swecker Jr, DVM, PhD   Robert J. Van Saun, DVM, MS, PhD
Editors

At one time or other, deficiencies of almost all of the essential nutrients have been considered to cause infertility in the cow.[1]

The quote, attributed to Meites in a book by T.J. McClure, is seminal to the objective of this issue on trace minerals. Although McClure's book is focused on nutrition and reproduction, the role of trace minerals is often brought into the conversation when the practitioner is trying to solve an acute or ongoing lack of productive or reproductive efficiency or an increase in infectious disease, especially when both management and ration appear to be adequate. Could it be the trace minerals? McClure went further to define both nutritional and metabolic infertility. Nutritional infertility is attributed to disorders where obvious clinical signs clearly point to a likely nutritional deficiency (eg, poor pregnancy rates in beef cows who calved in body condition score 3). This would be similar to a diagnosis of a classic trace element deficiency like white muscle disease associated with selenium deficiency. Clinical signs or necropsy findings point to a diagnosis. Metabolic infertility is considered when the animal does not show classic clinical signs, yet performance is below expectations. This parallel also works for trace minerals, as marginal or subclinical deficiencies have been associated with decreased production, increased disease occurrence via impaired immune function, or reproductive inefficiency. Even without decreased performance, trace mineral supplementation has a cost and should be delivered in a cost-effective manner.

Critical evaluation of trace mineral status involves the interpretation of multiple minerals, multiple interactions in the feed, water, and animal, and potential for toxicoses. Perhaps many veterinarians remember the complex wheel of interactions among the trace minerals that was presented in an undergraduate nutrition course. Our goal of this issue is to provide an overview of the role of trace minerals in ruminant health

Vet Clin Food Anim 39 (2023) xi–xii
https://doi.org/10.1016/j.cvfa.2023.08.011
0749-0720/23/© 2023 Published by Elsevier Inc.

and productivity, followed by nutritional and management strategies for multiple rumi-nant species within common production systems. We hope the practitioner is able to glean critical information from this issue to assure their clients have a functional yet cost-effective trace mineral program.

The issue editors are appreciative of the various article authors contributing to this collection. The scope of expertise is exceptional in addressing the many different pro-duction systems in which our ruminant animals are managed. One needs to remember that all trace mineral nutrition is geographically based; thus, there is no one trace mineral supplement template to apply to the various systems. More recent research has focused on trace mineral sources relative to bioavailability and ruminal interactions. We have attempted to address this scope of trace mineral metabolism, supplementa-tion, and diagnostics in a practical way allowing the practitioner to gain better insight into the challenges of trace mineral nutrition.

William S. Swecker Jr, DVM, PhD
Veterinary Teaching Hospital
Virginia–Maryland Regional College
of Veterinary Medicine
Virginia Tech
205 Duckpond Drive
Blacksburg, VA 24061-0442, USA

Robert J. Van Saun, DVM, MS, PhD
Department of Veterinary & Biomedical Sciences
College of Agricultural Sciences
Pennsylvania State University
108C Animal, Veterinary &
Biomedical Sciences Building
University Park, PA 16802-3500, USA

E-mail addresses:
cvmwss@vt.edu (W.S. Swecker)
rjv10@psu.edu (R.J. Van Saun)

REFERENCE

1. McClure TJ W. Nutritional and metabolic infertility in the cow. Wallingford: CAB In-ternational; 1994.

Trace Mineral Feeding and Assessment

William S. Swecker Jr, DVM, PhD

KEYWORDS

- Trace minerals • Supplementation • Assessment • Ruminants

KEY POINTS

- The trace minerals cobalt, copper, iodine, iron, manganese, molybdenum, selenium, and zinc are essential to the health of ruminant livestock.
- Trace minerals can be provided via multiple options.
- Classic trace mineral deficiencies should be eliminated by feeding recommended amounts unless antagonists are present.
- Advances in analytical technology allows for the accurate measurement of multiple trace minerals in a single small sample. Picking the correct sample, however, is equally important.
- Measurement of intake of trace mineral supplements in evaluation of the program.

INTRODUCTION AND OVERVIEW: TRACE MINERAL FUNCTION AND REQUIREMENTS, CONTENT OF COMMON FEEDS, AND ASSESSMENT OF THE FEEDS, SUPPLEMENTS, AND ANIMALS
Definition of an Essential Trace Mineral

The reader may find multiple definitions of trace minerals, with most referring to a minute concentration of functional minerals in animals or plants. From a nutritional perspective, however, an essential trace mineral should meet the following criteria.

1. Unique structure distinct from other nutrients
2. A function for that nutrient has been identified
3. A specific syndrome associated with deficiency has been identified.

Most references list eight trace minerals as essential for ruminants: copper (Cu), cobalt (Co), iron (Fe), iodine (I), manganese (Mn), molybdenum (Mo), selenium (Se), and zinc (Zn). The list may not be complete as researchers provide evidence that other trace minerals, like chromium, may have biologic function, but neither signs of deficiency or requirements have been determined.[1,2]

Virginia-Maryland Regional College of Veterinary Medicine, Virginia Tech, 205 Duckpond Drive, Blacksburg, VA 24061-0442, USA
E-mail address: cvmwss@vt.edu

Vet Clin Food Anim 39 (2023) 385–397
https://doi.org/10.1016/j.cvfa.2023.05.001
0749-0720/23/© 2023 Elsevier Inc. All rights reserved.

Within the required trace minerals, the requirements of Cu, Fe, Mn, and Zn are in the hundreds of milligrams/day where Co, I, and Se are required in mgs/day. This 50- to 100-fold difference is visually demonstrated in **Fig. 1** showing the relative requirements of the trace elements as compared to the macro minerals.

Functions of the Trace Elements

Most trace minerals function as components of enzymes (Cu, Mn, Mo, Se, Zn), components of vitamins (Co, I), or oxygen transport (Fe). These minerals may also serve as activators of enzyme systems, or some functions have yet to be determined. The known or common functions of the trace elements and deficiency signs are provided in **Table 1**.

Requirements

The requirements of a specific nutrient can be estimated by several methods, but the most common for production animals is the factorial approach which takes the amount needed to maintain the animal and then adds the requirement for additional factors like milk production, tissue growth, or fetal growth. The requirement for trace minerals is mg/animal/day in the factorial model, thus feeding guidelines convert the requirement to mg/kg diet while assuming normal intakes for that animal. The factorial model is preferred when the data are available. A nutrient response model is where varied concentrations of the nutrient are fed and responses are evaluated. This methodology has also contributed to the determination of trace mineral requirements. A challenge with the nutrient response model is which variable or variables should be used to determine the requirement? Should it be the minimal concentration that prevents a classic deficiency, the amount that maximizes enzyme function, or the amount

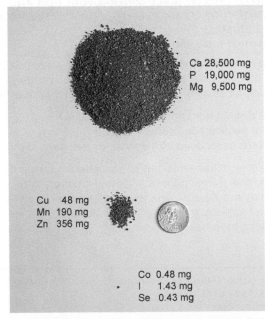

Ca 28,500 mg
P 19,000 mg
Mg 9,500 mg

Cu   48 mg
Mn 190 mg
Zn 356 mg

Co 0.48 mg
I   1.43 mg
Se 0.43 mg

Fig. 1. Representation of the dairy required amounts of macrominerals and trace minerals required for a 250-kg stressed beef calf, 0 to 14 days after arrival, Nutrient Requirements of Beef Cattle, 8th revised edition.

Table 1
Function and signs of deficiency for trace minerals required by ruminants

Mineral	Function	Classic Deficiency	Other Signs of Deficiency	Comments
Cobalt (Co)	Component of vitamin B12	Anemia	Decreased appetite and growth	Rumen microbes synthesize B12
Copper (Cu)	Lysyl oxidase, cytochrome oxidase, Cu, Zn superoxide dismutase (SOD1), ceruloplasmin, tyrosinase	Achromotrichia or gray hair on black cattle, enzootic ataxia in sheep	Decreased growth, decreased reproduction, decreased immune function	High Mo, Fe, and Sulfur can decrease Cu availability. Sheep are sensitive to toxicosis. Narrowest margin between meeting requirements and toxicosis
Iodine (I)	Component of thyroxine (T4) and triiodothyronine (T3)	Goiter	Hairless or weak calves, decreased reproduction in males and females	Goitrogens in some Brassica sp forages interfere with I absorption
Iron (Fe)	Hemoglobin, myoglobin, cytochromes, and Fe-S proteins in electron transport chain	Hypochromic, microcytic anemia	Decreased feed intake and weight gain	Deficiency unlikely unless chronic blood loss
Manganese (Mn)	Pyruvate carboxylase, arginase, Mn superoxide dismutase (SOD2). Activator for other enzymes	Reduced fertility, skeletal abnormalities in calves		Deficiencies rare
Molybdenum (Mo)	Xanthine oxidase, sulfite oxidase, aldehyde oxidase	Unknown		Increased Mo interferes with Cu
Selenium (Se)	Glutathione peroxidase, iodothyronine 5'-deiodinase	White muscle disease, Heinz body anemia	Weight loss, diarrhea, decreased immune function	
Zinc (Zn)	Cu-Zn superoxide dismutase, carbonic anhydrase, alkaline phosphatase, and others. Absorption of vitamin A	Parakeratotic lesions on skin. Decreased testicular growth.	Decreased growth, feed intake, and feed efficiency. Decreased immune function.	
Chromium (Cr)	Component of glucose tolerance factor			No requirement established at this time

that is associated with a desired production response like increased pregnancy rates? The reader can review the relevant nutrient requirements of the species in question to evaluate the data used to determine the specific trace mineral requirement.

Many of the foundation studies in determination of trace mineral requirements and digestibility were performed in the 1960s with the use of radioisotopes to determine both digestibility and distribution of the mineral within the body, and these studies still serve as a basis for many requirements today.[1,3]

For example, Miller states in a 1975 review that health and performance was reported to be normal when calves were fed purified diets with 9-ppm Zn.[4] Miller, however goes further to note that 20- to 40-ppm zinc in some diets was not sufficient for optimal performance. Miller notes that mild zinc deficiency may be expressed as decreases in intake, milk production, disease resistance, and reproductive function. As the reader can note in **Table 1**, decreased growth, reproduction, and immune function are associated with multiple trace minerals. Guyot and colleagues reported an epidemiologic study in Belgium where herds were classified as sick or healthy based on various pathologies observed in cows or calves, and Cu, I, Se, and Zn status of the cattle was measured.[5] The mean plasma Cu, plasma I, plasma Zn, and erythrocyte glutathione peroxidase (GPX) (Se) were lower in the sick herds, and 70% to 90% of the sick herds would be considered deficient in one or more trace minerals as compared to 0% to 10% of the healthy herds. Only 46% of the sick herds were offered mineral supplements as compared to 100% of the healthy herds. In the author's opinion, the current requirements will meet the needs to prevent classic deficiencies, yet the optimal amounts for enzyme function or production outcomes may be higher.

Conditionally Essential Nutrients

Over the past 20 years, the concept of conditionally essential nutrients has been developed. The concept is that nutrient requirements are determined on normal animals, yet there will be certain conditions, for example, stress or increased demands like pregnancy, where an additional supply is needed or is beneficial. As such, the recently weaned calf, the periparturient female, or external stressors like heat stress have been proposed as conditions where additional trace elements are needed.[6–9] This concept is expressed in the latest revision of Nutrient Requirements of Beef Cattle where the suggested nutrient concentrations for stressed calves are higher than the recommendations for other classes of beef cattle.[10] These suggestions are made with the understanding that feed intake of stressed calves is below that of unstressed calves and thus the increased concentrations compensate for the lack of intake. Conversely, the lactating female and growing animal increase their intake, thus the need for higher concentrations in the diet for those conditions is less clear, especially when the factorial model has been used to determine requirements.

Maximum Tolerable Concentrations

All the essential trace minerals have the potential to cause toxicoses, and many can antagonize the absorption of other minerals. Most nutrient requirement sources will also list maximum tolerable concentrations (MTCs), which is the amount that can still be safely fed to the animals in question. The MTC is usually 10× higher than the requirement, thus toxicosis are rare unless there is a mistake in formulation or the feed source is extremely high in one or more trace minerals. Copper, however, deserves special comment as it has the lowest difference between requirement and MTC, especially for sheep. Thus, the old adage, if a little is good, then more is better, should not be applied to trace mineral nutriture. The potential for bioaccumulation of the trace minerals to toxic concentrations is present and should be considered in nutrient management plans of intensive operations.[11]

Trace Mineral Content of Common Feeds

The soil content of the various minerals is a major determinant of the trace mineral content of the grain or forage grown on the soil. Regional differences in trace mineral concentration or risks of trace mineral deficiencies and toxicoses are reported in various regions of the United States.[12] For example, Se concentrations tend to be high in the upper Great Plains but low in the coastal regions. However, large variations in trace mineral content can also be noted within regions or states.[12] The reader can access the National Geochemical Survey to get an overview of soil trace mineral content in their region of the United States: https://mrdata.usgs.gov/geochem/method. php. An example of the concentration of trace mineral concentration of legume hay, grass hay, and corn silage analyzed at the Dairy One Laboratory, Ithaca, NY, is shown in **Fig. 2**.

Cu and Zn concentrations in common forages are commonly inadequate to meet the needs of beef cattle, while Fe concentrations are rarely inadequate, and many samples contain concentrations above MTCs. A minimum requirement for Mo has not been defined; thus, no feeds would be considered deficient in Mo. Even if concentrations do not exceed MTC, high concentrations may antagonize the absorption of other minerals, for example, high Fe and Mo depress Cu absorption. Laboratory analysis of the trace mineral content of commonly used feeds is recommended to give the best representation of trace mineral intake from supplied feeds.

Grazing ruminants will consume soil as part of the grazing process as the soil is present on the surface of the plant or the ruminant may directly consume soil in a process known as geophagy. Researchers have estimated that soil intake is usually 1% to 2% of dry matter intake in grazing ruminants but can be much higher.[13,14] Harvested feeds like hay and silage will also have some level of soil present but is dependent on cutting height and harvest method. The actual consumption of soil, also known as geophagy, by domestic or wild ruminants is a commonly observed process, but the instinct or drive behind geophagy is poorly understood. Lavelle and colleagues reported that sodium content of soil was associated with geophagy in wild cervids but data were lacking to support the concept of "mineral wisdom" or that domestic ruminants eat soil to correct specific trace mineral deficiencies.[15]

Supplementation Methods

Common methods of trace mineral supplementation include (1) provision of trace minerals in a total mixed ration (TMR), (2) a limit-fed protein or energy supplement with trace minerals, (3) a free-choice salt-macromineral-trace mineral mixture in block or loose form, (4) free-choice trace mineral salt in block or loose form, or (5) pulse dosing by drench, paste, or injection. The advantages of the TMR and limit-fed supplement are obvious as the intake is consistent and repeatable; thus, there should be limited variation among animals fed the same ration. In addition, animals with higher production, either lactation or growth, increase intake to support that production.

The Association of American Feed Control Officials (AAFCO) does provide species-specific guidance for mineral supplements and feeds. The following list provides an example for beef mineral feeds.[16]

Beef cattle feed—mineral supplements
a. A minimum and maximum guarantee for calcium
b. A minimum guarantee for phosphorus

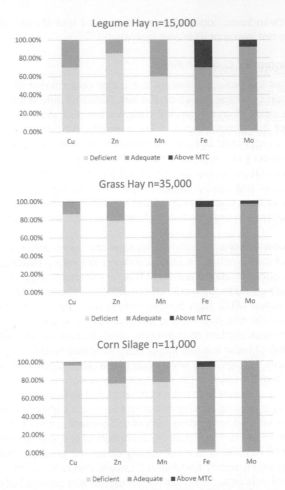

Fig. 2. Classification of forage trace mineral content of legume hay, grass hay, and corn silage samples relative to the nutrient requirements of gestating beef cows from the Nutrient Requirements of Beef Cattle, 8th revised edition. Forages were analyzed by the Dairy One Forage Laboratory, Ithaca, NY. MTC, maximum tolerable concentration (the concentration that can be safely fed to the beef cattle).

c. A minimum and maximum guarantee for salt, if added
d. A minimum and maximum guarantee for total sodium, if total sodium exceeds that furnished by the maximum salt guarantee
e. A minimum guarantee for magnesium
f. A minimum guarantee for potassium
g. A minimum guarantee for copper in parts per million (ppm)
h. A minimum guarantee for selenium in parts per million (ppm)
i. A minimum guarantee for zinc in parts per million (ppm)
j. A minimum guarantee for vitamin A, other than precursors of vitamin A, in international units per pound, if added.

Critical evaluation of labels is essential to correctly determine what is being fed as there are no defined standards on the amount of any given mineral in a product other than the AAFCO definition of iodized salt which states, "Iodized Salt, is a common salt (NaCl) containing not less than 0.007% iodine."[17]

Intake of Free-Choice Products

Many salt-mineral products are available in block and loose forms; however, there are limited data on individual animal consumption of these products, partially due to the technical difficulties in obtaining the data. Rocks and colleagues reported that the consumption of loose salt by sheep was 2- to 7-fold higher than that of salt blocks.[18] Morris reported an average consumption of 27 g/day for beef cows offered salt blocks.[19] Although not a direct comparison, other authors have reported consumption rates of 50 to 200 g/day of loose salt-mineral mixtures.[20–24] Based on these studies, consumption of a mineral mix in loose form is greater than that in block form.

Salt concentration is a major driver of intake as ruminants appear to have an appetite for salt. Although ruminants may select different macromineral sources depending on the current diet,[25] they do not appear to have the ability to correct deficiencies for the various macrominerals or trace minerals as promoted by the "buffet approach" with each mineral offered separately.[26,27] Feed companies will add minor amounts of grains or flavoring agents to salt-mineral mixtures to promote intake. It is the author's opinion that cattle will acclimate to specific flavors and thus voluntarily depress intake when a different mineral is offered.

Most producers can produce a label with the concentrations of the various trace minerals offered to the animals. Measurement of intake, however, is not commonly done in the author's experience, and like any ration, intake × consumption = nutrient supply to the animal. It is critical with free-choice products to have some measure of intake to evaluate the risk of trace mineral deficiencies or excesses.

Pulse-Dosed Products: Injectables, Drenches, Pastes, and boluses

Another option for trace mineral supplementation is to provide each animal trace minerals through injection, drenching, pastes, or boluses. To the authors knowledge, there are only 2 trace mineral products that have gone through an FDA approval process: iron dextran and sodium selenite. Many of the currently marketed products have been used around periods of high stress like calving and weaning or in an effort to improve pregnancy rates at breeding. Rapid increases in the various trace minerals were noted within hours to days on either blood or liver parameters, but the increase tended to only last days to weeks.[28–30] Pulse dosing would appear to be most useful when there is a known deficiency or risk of deficiency (eg, purchased stocker calves from specific regions) to provide an immediate supply of trace minerals. The pulsed dose should be followed by adequate supplementation in the feed or mineral mix.

Assessing Adequacy

Interpretation of the trace mineral status can involve analysis of the animal, the feed, water, or all three. Clark and Ellison suggested that the approach to testing for mineral adequacy in animals should first take into consideration the question that is being asked.[31] They define 4 categories to consider.

1. Is poor performance due to a trace mineral deficiency?
2. Are animals on the farm at risk of deficiency?
3. Do animals have adequate reserves of trace minerals before going into a period where demand is increasing or supply is decreasing?
4. Is the supplementation program adequate?

Who Should Be Sampled?

A first step in analysis would be to consider which animals should be sampled based on the question being asked? As an example, if the question is around poor performance, then the animals to be sampled should be average representatives of the poor-performing group. An obvious temptation is to sample the worst-looking animal(s) in the pen or the animal who has been given the most antibiotic treatments. Don't do it (**Fig. 3**)!

Chronic infection and depressed intake deplete trace minerals; thus, one should expect deficiencies in chronically ill animals. This challenge is not unique to production medicine; it is also common in human medicine in determination of mineral status of critically ill children.[32] To determine if the farm is at risk of deficiency, sample the animals with the highest demands, such as late gestation/early lactation females or rapidly growing calves, kids, or lambs. To determine if adequate reserves are present, sample groups prior to the increase in demand or decreased supply, for example, sample cows from cow-calf pairs prior to movement to an extensive summer pasture where supply of mineral is limited. To determine the adequacy of a supplementation program, sample the same animals before supplementation begins and during the supplementation period.

What tissue should be sampled on the animals?

Consultation with the diagnostic laboratory prior to sampling is valuable in assuring the correct sample is placed in the correct container and shipping conditions are optimized for accurate results. Reference intervals and analytical methodologies can differ between laboratories; thus, caution is advised when comparing results among laboratories. Individual animal results can be both interesting and confusing; thus, comparisons of the means of 5 to 15 animals are the best approach to develop conclusions of the herd's status.[31,33]

Measure the mineral or an enzyme?

The biologic functions of trace minerals are related to an enzyme, vitamin, or hormone that contains that trace mineral; thus, the measurement of the mineral itself is a proxy for function. The use of enzyme assays tend to be restricted to research studies as

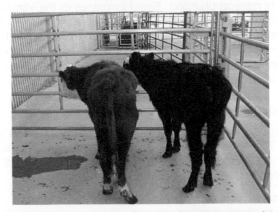

Fig. 3. Two calves presented for evaluation for lack of response to multiple antibiotic treatments for bovine respiratory disease complex. These calves would not be a good choice for trace mineral assessment as they are likely deficient in one or more minerals due to chronic disease and anorexia.

enzymes are less stable and most assays have not been cross-validated among laboratories.[34] The adoption of inductively coupled plasma-source mass spectrometry for the analysis of trace minerals in biological matrixes now allows diagnostic laboratories to analyze one small plasma or liver sample for multiple minerals.[35,36] Mineral concentrations, rather than enzyme assays, are most commonly used for diagnostic purposes.

Which tissue?

The practitioner has the option of sampling whole blood, plasma/serum, liver, or hair, and there are advantages and disadvantages to each sample. Whole-blood analysis should be restricted to Se as the majority of Se is in the red blood cell in the form of glutathione peroxidase; thus, hemolysis during collection or storage is not an issue.[37] Plasma is a convenient and tempting sample, especially at the herd level and can be helpful in diagnosing severe deficiencies of Cu and Zn, but is not as sensitive and specific to determine marginal status.[38,39] Serum concentrations of both Cu and Zn can change during periods of stress. For example, VanValin and colleagues reported greater than 50% decline in plasma zinc 6 hours after administration of lipopolysaccharide (LPS) to Angus-cross steers, but concentrations returned to preinjection concentrations within 48 hours.[40] Laboratories may request that serum or plasma samples for Zn analysis should be placed in special trace element tubes due to potential Zn contamination in the classic red top tube; however, that finding has recently been challenged with the suggestion that red top tubes are acceptable.[41] Hussein and colleagues reported that the use of heparin or ethylenediaminetetraacetic acid as an anticoagulant influenced the plasma concentrations of Cu, Se, and Mn when compared to each other and serum.[42] They did note a strong correlation between pooling 8 samples and pooling individual samples; thus, pooling of samples may be a reasonable option to decrease costs of sampling and analysis.

Liver biopsies have been considered the gold standard for evaluation of trace element status of ruminants. The advent of analytical techniques to detect multiple minerals on a small biopsy sample has allowed the use of smaller biopsy tools like a 16-gauge biopsy tool.[36] The biopsy sample can be obtained via a percutaneous route on the right side of the animal.[43,44] Liver samples can also be collected from dead animals including abortions, stillbirths, and perinatal deaths with adjustments made for the age of the fetus or calf.[45,46]

Hair is an intriguing sample for analysis of biologic compounds as the compound is deposited at the level of the hair follicle during growth; thus, the analysis of hair could also provide a temporal pattern, for example, the hair closest to the body reflects recent status, and hair farther from the body would represent past status. Hair may be useful in the analysis of cortisol in stress studies[47] or exposure to toxic heavy metals like lead or cadmium[48] but do not appear, at this time, to be a reasonable or effective sample in assessing the trace mineral status of livestock.[49] Contamination by soil or manure, processing and cleaning of the sample, breed, and hair color all are challenges in interpretation of hair trace mineral concentration.[50]

Feed analysis

Feed sampling has its own challenges, and one key element is getting a representative sample of the feedstuff. For hays, it is taking core samples from at least 10 bales. For silages, it is taking multiple samples from the silo face, mixing them, and then subsampling from the mixture. Even when sampling a mineral mixture, correct sampling via a corer or mixing of the entire bag prior to sampling is needed rather than taking a handful out of the top of the bag. The author has observed that feed analysis is underutilized, and a common response to a deficiency case is to pulse dose or add supplemental trace minerals to the ration without knowing what is in the basal ration. Feed analysis will reveal which feed or feeds are deficient or which feed or feeds contain high concentrations of antagonists. Changing the feed sources can be a valuable and simpler long-term option, at times, rather than changing the supplemental trace minerals.

Interpretation of Results

For trace elements, diagnostic labs may use the terms deficient, marginal, adequate, and high/toxic. There are no international definitions of these terms, but consider the following guideline.

1. Deficient: classic clinical signs of trace mineral deficiency are associated with this concentration. Additional supplementation is beneficial.
2. Marginal: classic clinical signs are usually not evident, but the performance may be impaired or the herd is at risk of deficiencies. Additional supplementation may help.
3. Adequate: concentrations are similar to animals that have been fed adequate concentrations of the mineral in question. Additional supplementation is not needed, and supplementation may be decreased if concentrations are on the high end of the adequate range.
4. High/toxic: concentrations are associated with signs of toxicosis, and supplementation of this mineral should be limited or removed.

SUMMARY

Trace minerals are a required component of an animal's diet. The clinical presentations of deficient and marginal status can be as broad as decreased growth or reproduction or very specific like white muscle disease or achromotrichia. If trace element deficiencies or excesses are on the rule-out list for the problem at hand, then sampling the animals is a reasonable first step. The next steps are to evaluate the concentrations of the trace elements in feeds and supplements and the intake of feed and supplements. The practitioner is encouraged to establish a relationship with a diagnostic laboratory to become familiar with the common deficiencies in their practice region as well as determination of the best sampling techniques to evaluate the trace mineral status of the animals under their care.

DISCLOSURE

The authors have nothing to disclose.

REFERENCES

1. Miller WJ. New Concepts and Developments in Metabolism and Homeostasis of Inorganic Elements in Dairy Cattle. A Review. J Dairy Sci 1975;58(10):1549–60.
2. Spears JW, Whisnant CS, Huntington GB, et al. Chromium propionate enhances insulin sensitivity in growing cattle. J Dairy Sci 2012;95(4):2037–45.
3. Miller JK. New techniques for intensive research with dairy cattle–mineral research. J Dairy Sci 1972;55(8):1211–9.
4. Miller WJ. Zinc Nutrition of Cattle: A Review. J Dairy Sci 1970;53(8):1123–35.
5. Guyot H, Saegerman C, Lebreton P, et al. Epidemiology of trace elements deficiencies in Belgian beef and dairy cattle herds. J Trace Elem Med Biol 2009; 23(2):116–23.

6. Ogilvie L, Spricigo JFW, Mion B, et al. Neutrophil function and antibody production during the transition period: Effect of form of supplementary trace minerals and associations with postpartum clinical disease and blood metabolites. J Dairy Sci 2022;105(12):9944–60.

7. Moriel P, Arthington JD. Effects of trace mineral-fortified, limit-fed preweaning supplements on performance of pre- and postweaned beef calves. J Anim Sci 2013;91(3):1371–80.

8. Weng X, Monteiro APA, Guo J, et al. Effects of heat stress and dietary zinc source on performance and mammary epithelial integrity of lactating dairy cows. J Dairy Sci 2018;101(3):2617–30.

9. Silva TH, Guimaraes I, Menta PR, et al. Effect of injectable trace mineral supplementation on peripheral polymorphonuclear leukocyte function, antioxidant enzymes, health, and performance in dairy cows in semi-arid conditions. J Dairy Sci 2022;105(2):1649–60.

10. National Academies of Sciences E, Medicine. Nutrient requirements of beef cattle. 8th Revised Edition. Washington, DC: The National Academies Press; 2016.

11. Brugger D, Windisch WM. Environmental responsibilities of livestock feeding using trace mineral supplements. Anim Nutr 2015;1(3):113–8.

12. Berger LL. Variation in the Trace Mineral Content of Feedstuffs. Prof Anim Sci 1996;12(1):1–5.

13. Thornton I, Abrahams P. Soil ingestion — a major pathway of heavy metals into livestock grazing contaminated land. Sci Total Environ 1983;28(1):287–94.

14. Fries GF, Marrow GS, Snow PA. Soil ingestion by dairy cattle. J Dairy Sci 1982; 65(4):611–8.

15. Lavelle MJ, Phillips GE, Fischer JW, et al. Mineral licks: motivational factors for visitation and accompanying disease risk at communal use sites of elk and deer. Environ Geochem Health 2014;36(6):1049–61.

16. Officials AoAFC. Animal feed labeling guide. Champaign, IL: Association of American Feed Control Officials; 2020.

17. Officials AoAFC. Official Publication Association of American Feed Control Officials Incorporated, 2021.

18. Rocks R, Wheeler J, Hedges D. Labelled waters of crystallization in gypsum to measure the intake by sheep of loose and compressed mineral supplements. Aust J Exp Agric 1982;22(115):35–42.

19. Morris JG, Delmas RE, Hull JL. Salt (Sodium) Supplementation of Range Beef Cows in California. J Anim Sci 1980;51(3):722–31.

20. Patterson JD, Burris WR, Boling JA, et al. Individual Intake of Free-Choice Mineral Mix by Grazing Beef Cows May Be Less Than Typical Formulation Assumptions and Form of Selenium in Mineral Mix Affects Blood Se Concentrations of Cows and Their Suckling Calves. Biol Trace Elem Res 2013;155(1):38–48.

21. Pehrson B, Ortman K, Madjid N, et al. The influence of dietary selenium as selenium yeast or sodium selenite on the concentration of selenium in the milk of Suckler cows and on the selenium status of their calves. J Anim Sci 1999; 77(12):3371–6.

22. Swecker WS Jr, eversole DE, Thatcher CD, et al. Selenium Supplementation of Gestating Beef Cows on Selenium-Deficient Pastures. Agri Pract 1991;12(2): 25–30.

23. Arthington JD, Silveira ML, Caramalac LS, et al. Effects of varying sources of Cu, Zn, and Mn on mineral status and preferential intake of salt-based supplements by beef cows and calves and rainfall-induced metal loss. Transl Anim Sci 2021; 5(2):txab046.

24. Cockwill C, McAllister T, Olson M, et al. Individual intake of mineral and molasses supplements by cows, heifers and calves. Canadian Journal of Animal Science - CAN J ANIM SCI 2000;80:681–90.

25. Villalba JJ, Provenza FD, Hall JO. Learned appetites for calcium, phosphorus, and sodium in sheep1,2. J Anim Sci 2008;86(3):738–47.

26. Muller LD, Schaffer LV, Ham LC, et al. Cafeteria Style Free-Choice Mineral Feeder for Lactating Dairy-Cows. J Dairy Sci 1977;60(10):1574–82.

27. Zervas G, Rissaki M, Deligeorgis S. Free-choice consumption of mineral lick blocks by fattening lambs fed ad libitum alfalfa hay and concentrates with different trace mineral content. Livest Prod Sci 2001;68(2):251–8.

28. Swecker WS Jr, Hunter KH, Shanklin RK, et al. Parenteral selenium and vitamin E supplementation of weaned beef calves. J Vet Intern Med/American College of Veterinary Internal Medicine 2008;22(2):443–9.

29. Jackson TD, Carmichael RN, Deters EL, et al. Comparison of multiple single-use, pulse-dose trace mineral products provided as injectable, oral drench, oral paste, or bolus on circulating and liver trace mineral concentrations of beef steers. Applied Animal Science 2020;36(1):26–35.

30. Pogge DJ, Richter EL, Drewnoski ME, et al. Mineral concentrations of plasma and liver after injection with a trace mineral complex differ among Angus and Simmental cattle. J Anim Sci 2012;90(8):2692–8.

31. Clark RG, Ellison RS. Mineral testing–the approach depends on what you want to find out. N Z Vet J 1993;41(2):98–100.

32. Dao DT, Anez-Bustillos L, Cho BS, et al. Assessment of Micronutrient Status in Critically Ill Children: Challenges and Opportunities. Nutrients 2017;9(11).

33. Laven RA, Nortje R. Diagnosis of the Cu and Se status of dairy cattle in New Zealand: How many samples are needed? N Z Vet J 2013;61(5):269–73.

34. Lum GE, Rowntree JE, Bondioli KR, et al. The influence of dietary selenium on common indicators of selenium status and liver glutathione peroxidase-1 messenger ribonucleic acid. J Anim Sci 2009;87(5):1739–46.

35. Ward NI, Abou-Shakra FR, Durrant SF. Trace elemental content of biological materials. Biol Trace Elem Res 1990;26(1):177–87.

36. Radke SL, Ensley SM, Hansen SL. Inductively coupled plasma mass spectrometry determination of hepatic copper, manganese, selenium, and zinc concentrations in relation to sample amount and storage duration. J Vet Diagn Invest 2020; 32(1):103–7.

37. Scholz RW, Hutchinson LJ. Distribution of glutathione peroxidase activity and selenium in the blood of dairy cows. Am J Vet Res 1979;40(2):245–9.

38. Minatel L, Carfagnini JC. Evaluation of the diagnostic value of plasma copper levels in cattle. Prev Vet Med 2002;53(1–2):1–5.

39. Claypool DW, Adams FW, Pendell HW, et al. Relationship between the level of copper in the blood plasma and liver of cattle. J Anim Sci 1975;41(3):911–4.

40. VanValin KR, Carmichael-Wyatt RN, Deters EL, et al. Dietary zinc concentration and lipopolysaccharide injection affect circulating trace minerals, acute phase protein response, and behavior as evaluated by an ear-tag-based accelerometer in beef steers. J Anim Sci 2021;99(10):skab278.

41. Love M, Laven RA. Measurement of serum zinc concentration in ruminants: a comparison of results from standard serum and specific trace element collection tubes. N Z Vet J 2020;68(6):349–52.

42. Hussein HA, Müller AE, Staufenbiel R. Comparative evaluation of mineral profiles in different blood specimens of dairy cows at different production phases. Front Vet Sci 2022;9:905249.

43. Smart ME, Northcote MJ. Liver Biopsies in Cattle. Compend Continuing Educ Pract Vet 1985;7(5):S327–32.
44. Swecker WS. Trace Mineral Feeding and Assessment. Vet Clin Food Anim Pract 2014. https://doi.org/10.1016/j.cvfa.2014.07.008.
45. Factors Influencing Bovine Maternal and Fetal Hepatic Mineral Concentrations. 13th International Conference on Production Diseases in Farm Animals; 2007. Meeting held in 7/29/2007 to 8/4/2007, Leipzig, Germany.
46. Waldner CL, Blakley B. Evaluating micronutrient concentrations in liver samples from abortions, stillbirths, and neonatal and postnatal losses in beef calves. J Vet Diagn Invest 2014;26(3):376–89.
47. Tallo-Parra O, Manteca X, Sabes-Alsina M, et al. Hair cortisol detection in dairy cattle by using EIA: protocol validation and correlation with faecal cortisol metabolites. Animal 2015;9(6):1059–64.
48. Patra RC, Swarup D, Sharma MC, et al. Trace mineral profile in blood and hair from cattle environmentally exposed to lead and cadmium around different industrial units. J Vet Med 2006;53(10):511–7.
49. Spears JW, Brandao VLN, Heldt J. Invited Review: Assessing trace mineral status in ruminants, and factors that affect measurements of trace mineral status. Applied Animal Science 2022;38(3):252–67.
50. Combs DK, Goodrich RD, Meiske JC. Mineral concentrations in hair as indicators of mineral status: a review. J Anim Sci 1982;54(2):391–8.

Trace Mineral Metabolism
The Maternal-Fetal Bond

Robert J. Van Saun, DVM, MS, PhD

KEYWORDS

- Trace minerals • Transition metabolism • Fetal metabolism • Ruminant

KEY POINTS

- The fetal liver is capable to storing trace minerals obtained from maternal nutrient transfer to concentrations that exceed those of the maternal liver without inducing toxicosis.
- Both placental and colostral transfer of minerals is dependent upon maternal mineral status.
- Interpretation of measured hepatic mineral content of a fetus, neonate, and adult animal is confounded by changing moisture content with increasing age, thus requiring age-based criteria.
- Liver is the primary trace mineral storage pool in the body that supports maintenance of essential physiologic functions in the presence of dietary mineral inadequacies and best reflects nutritive status.

INTRODUCTION

Minerals, both macrominerals and microminerals, have many important biologic roles and are essential nutrients. The macrominerals calcium, phosphorus, magnesium, sodium, potassium, chloride, and sulfur are associated with skeletal structure, acid-base balance (electrolytes in blood), plasma membrane potentials, and energy metabolism.[1] Most macrominerals are homeostatically regulated to various degrees. In contrast, microminerals (ie, trace minerals) cobalt (Co), copper (Cu), iodine (I), iron (Fe), manganese (Mn), selenium (Se), and zinc (Zn) play many roles in metabolic regulation, metabolic reactions via various metalloenzymes, immune function, and antioxidant capacity (see Swecker, 2023).[1] Unlike macrominerals, trace minerals are not homeostatically regulated but through either modification of intestinal uptake efficiency or renal excretion and movement between physiologic-defined pools.[1,2] Trace minerals have been implicated in various clinical disease conditions associated with

Department of Veterinary and Biomedical Sciences, College of Agricultural Sciences, Pennsylvania State University, 108C Animal, Veterinary and Biomedical Sciences Building, University Park, PA 16802-3500, USA
E-mail address: rjv10@psu.edu

Vet Clin Food Anim 39 (2023) 399–412
https://doi.org/10.1016/j.cvfa.2023.06.003
0749-0720/23/© 2023 Elsevier Inc. All rights reserved.

vetfood.theclinics.com

either deficient or toxicosis status; however, there is much interest in their potential role in early embryonic and fetal development and postnatal survival.[3]

Surveys comparing abattoir and diagnostic lab fetal liver mineral concentrations have shown a significantly lower mineral concentrations in aborted fetuses (**Table 1**).[4,5] The question is whether the observed differences are a consequence or cause of fetal abortion. Graham and colleagues suggested the hepatic mineral differences were a consequence of abortion. Orr and Blakely described histologic lesions consistent with Se deficiency in aborted fetuses indicating a direct nutritional link.[6] Reported diagnostic outcomes for ruminant fetal abortion and stillbirth cases have been less than 45% when focused on microbiologic (ie, infectious), congenital, and traumatic etiologies.[7–10] This low diagnostic efficiency suggests existence of other potential etiologies, including nutritional deficiencies or toxicities.[11] A potential role for trace minerals in these pregnancy wastage outcomes has been suggested although confirmatory controlled feeding studies have not been performed.[4,6,12–14] The objective of this article is to describe the mineral interactions between the pregnant dam and her fetus as it potentially impacts fetal and early neonatal health and survival.

TRACE MINERAL METABOLISM OVERVIEW

Although not regulated via some homeostatic mechanism, body trace mineral balance is coordinated to ensure associated physiologic functions are maintained while the mineral-specific status is sustained. A simplified characterization of trace mineral physiology has used a three-pool model.[1,15] The biochemical function pool represents specific biologic roles of a trace mineral as a component of or cofactor to one or more metalloenzymes. Trace minerals being pro-oxidants need to be transported on blood carrier proteins or albumin, and this represents the transport mineral pool moving trace minerals throughout the body. Trace minerals are hepatically stored as metal complexes (ie, storage pool), and this pool is most sensitive to nutritional status.[16] If absorbed trace mineral uptake exceeds the requirement, minerals can be hepatically stored until other regulatory processes, reduced absorptive efficiency or increased renal excretion, modify net mineral retention back into balance. The transport pool is dynamic in reflecting changes relative to deficient or sufficient nutritive state, although buffered by mineral storage mobilization.[17] In mineral inadequacy, hepatic storage will be mobilized to maintain biochemical pool activity until absorptive efficiency, reduced excretion, or both can be enacted to raise net mineral retention.

Clinical trace mineral deficiency disease is then defined as a critical loss of some specific activity within the biochemical pool disrupting normal physiologic function.

Table 1
Comparison of fetal liver mineral concentrations (μg/g dry weight) in abattoir and diagnostic lab abortion samples from surveys completed in California (Graham et al., 1994) and Pennsylvania (Van Saun, 2010)[4,5]

Mineral	California		Pennsylvania	
	Abattoir	Abortion	Abattoir	Abortion
Copper (Cu)	438.3	207.3	403.6	253.2
Iron (Fe)	1402.5	700.6	1110.9	748.1
Manganese (Mn)	9.19	3.29	6.02	4.0
Selenium (Se)	ND	ND	2.6	1.5
Zinc (Zn)	927	359.4	807.6	414.0

For example, in clinical copper deficiency, the sign of achromotrichia is a consequence of inadequate melanin production due to loss of Cu-dependent tyrosinase activity.[1] Selenium-deficiency-associated muscle lesions (eg, white muscle disease) is associated with reduced Se-dependent glutathione peroxidase activity.[1] Trace mineral toxicosis is generally a result of pro-oxidative reactions. Subclinical disease is a consequence of marginal deficiency or toxicosis often presenting as impaired immune function, reduced growth rate, reproductive efficiency, or other nonspecific declines in productive efficiency. In using this simplified trace mineral physiology model, one must consider whether the interrelationships between mineral pools are the same for fetus, neonate, and adult in supporting basic body metabolism, development, and productivity.

Maternal Mineral Metabolism

Pregnancy trace mineral requirements are the sum of maintenance and pregnancy needs as well as maternal growth in the case of first-time pregnant dams. Models to estimate trace mineral requirements to support pregnancy are limited for most ruminants often resulting in recommendations for dietary concentration rather than a specified amount. House and Bell described bovine fetal mineral accretion during the last 3 months of pregnancy to estimate dairy cattle trace mineral pregnancy feeding recommendations.[18,19] Maintenance trace mineral requirement is the largest component of total requirement and the most variable one. Maintenance requirements are associated with dry matter intake, a function of body weight.[20–22] Pregnancy-specific trace mineral requirements for domestic ruminants are modeled after expected birth weight of fetus(es).[20–22]

Maternal nutrients available to the fetus would include those from the consumed diet as well as mobilized reserves, if needed. Maternal mineral transport pool delivers mineral resources to the interface of maternal and fetal placental components. Placental mineral transport mechanisms are not well characterized as the focus has been primarily on transfer of glucose and amino acids as these are the primary conceptus (ie, fetus and placenta) energy substrates.[23,24] Based on fetal hepatic mineral concentrations, most minerals are efficiently transferred to the fetus with exceptions of iodine and manganese.[25–28] Goiter due to iodine deficiency can be seen in aborted or stillborn fetuses without clinical signs of goiter in the dam.[1,29] Nutrient adequacy of the maternal diet will determine the extent of fetal hepatic mineral accretion and storage. Upregulation of Cu regulatory gene products in the fetal liver when the dam was fed a Cu-deficient diet suggests some level of fetal compensation when facing deficiency of a nutrient.[30]

In addition to placental mineral transfer throughout gestation, trace minerals are transferred into colostrum during the last weeks of gestation. Colostrum differs from milk as it contains greater trace mineral concentrations than milk (**Table 2**). Blood nutrient concentrations, namely fat-soluble vitamins and minerals, decline just prior to calving, suggesting significant transfer to colostrum, and this decline is attenuated with mastectomy.[31,32] Maternal hepatic and serum Se concentrations were lower during the last month of gestation in beef and dairy cattle suggestive of losses to colostrum.[33] Not all studies observed a decline in maternal mineral status with advancing gestation, possibly a result of differences in level of supplementation.[18,19] Maternal mineral losses during gestation to conceptus and colostrum, especially coupled with reduced or interrupted dietary supplementation during late gestation, might lead to compromised maternal nutritional status, resulting in compromised immune function and antioxidant capacity, thus predisposing the dam to periparturient diseases.[34]

Table 2
Comparison of calf mineral requirements with whole milk and colostrum mineral content

Mineral	Units	Calf Requirement[a]	Whole Milk[b]	Colostrum[b]
Total solids	g/100 g	100	13	12.5	23.9
Calcium	g/100 g	1.0	0.13	0.12	0.26
Phosphorus	g/100 g	0.70	0.09	0.10	0.17
Magnesium	g/100 g	0.07	0.009	0.01	0.04
Potassium	g/100 g	0.65	0.085	0.115	0.14
Sodium	g/100 g	0.40	0.052	0.05–0.15	0.07–0.14
Copper	mg/kg	10	1.3	0.15	0.39–0.6
Iron	mg/kg	100	13	0.05	0.2–2.0
Manganese	mg/kg	40	5.2	0.004	0.02–0.09
Selenium	mg/kg	0.3	0.039	0.005–0.03	0.04–0.056
Zinc	mg/kg	40	5.2	0.30	1.2–17.2

[a] Requirements shown on dry matter (100% total solids) and as-fed (13% total solids) basis.
[b] Whole milk and colostrum nutrient content on as-fed basis.
Adapted from NASEM, 2021.[21]

Fetal Mineral Metabolism

The developing fetus is totally dependent upon availability of essential nutrients from maternal blood via placental transfer. As a result, fetal nutrient status is reflective of maternal nutritive status. Maternal nutrient status, primarily the macronutrients, can have long-term impacts on fetal development and neonatal performance through modifications of genetic regulation (ie, fetal programming). The potential role of maternal mineral status on fetal and neonatal genetic programming is limited although recently reviewed.[35] Many studies have observed the ability of all minerals to concentrate in fetal liver while finding fetal hepatic mineral concentrations to exceed maternal values when compared on a dry matter basis.[25,26,28,33,36] Many laboratories report hepatic mineral concentrations on a wet weight basis, which masks concentrated fetal mineral concentrations as a result of lower dry matter content of the fetal liver. The mean fetal hepatic dry matter ratio was less (0.205 ± 0.02 vs. 0.242 ± 0.03, $P < .0001$) than neonatal hepatic dry matter ratio, and both means were lower (0.325 ± 0.03, $P < .0001$) than maternal dry matter ratio.[37] Hepatic dry matter ratio increased ($P < .0001$) with increasing fetal and postnatal age.[37]

Using paired maternal and associated fetal hepatic mineral concentrations determined in abattoir samples (n = 185), a ratio between fetal and maternal hepatic mineral concentration was calculated on a dry matter basis. Fetal-to-maternal mineral ratios were greater than 1, indicating greater hepatic mineral concentration in the fetus than in the dam, for Cu, Fe, Se, and Zn, while ratios for Mn, Mo, and Co were less than one.[38] Interestingly, when hepatic maternal-to-fetal mineral concentration ratios were calculated, maternal-fetal Cu ratio was also greater than 1; otherwise they were the opposite of what was determined for the fetal-maternal ratio.[38] The determined correlation between maternal and fetal hepatic mineral concentrations are quite insignificant[4,38]; however, when fetal-to-maternal ratio was plotted against maternal hepatic mineral concentration, there were more significant relationships for most minerals than with a direct comparison (**Fig. 1**). What these models suggest is a greater fetal hepatic mineral uptake in the face of low maternal mineral status and lower uptake

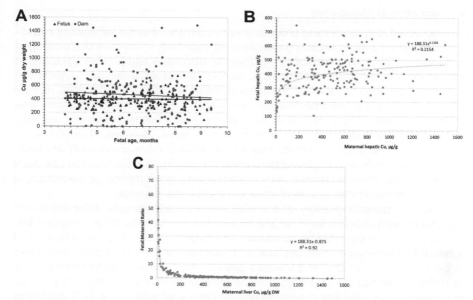

Fig. 1. Comparisons of dairy and beef cattle fetal and maternal hepatic copper (Cu) concentration (dry weight basis) in abattoir samples (n=185): Fetal and maternal hepatic Cu concentrations compared across gestational age (*A*), plot of fetal hepatic Cu concentration by maternal Cu concentration (*B*), and fetal-to-maternal ratio plotted by maternal hepatic Cu concentration (*C*).

when maternal mineral status was elevated. This relationship may explain the fetus' ability to concentrate minerals in the face of maternal deficiency yet protect against potential toxicity with maternal mineral excess.

Returning fetal blood from the placenta enters the fetus via the umbilical vein where the fetal liver is the first tissue to receive the nutrient-rich blood. The fetal liver clears most of the blood mineral, although the mechanisms are not understood, as fetal serum mineral concentrations are generally lower than maternal blood mineral concentrations.[33,39] The mean maternal serum Se concentration was twice that of her fetus; however, whole blood and erythrocyte Se concentrations were not different between the fetus and dam.[33] The mean whole blood glutathione peroxidase activity was only slightly greater in the fetus than that in the dam, which may be consistent with the higher fetal metabolic rate.[33] Other studies have also shown minimal differences between nonhepatic fetal tissue mineral concentrations and maternal tissue mineral concentrations.[27,28]

Observed differences between serum and liver Se concentrations suggest altered transport and storage pools between a dam and fetus. Although similar relationships have not been completely identified for other trace elements, similar mechanisms are thought to be in place given lower fetal serum mineral concentrations. A higher maternal serum mineral concentration provides a substantial concentration gradient necessary for efficient placental transport, assuming a lack of active transport mechanisms. Greater fetal hepatic mineral concentrations infer a preferential mineral storage over and above tissue requirements. Given these relationships, fetal liver and serum mineral concentrations must be interpreted differently from adult values. Nutrient-specific enzyme activity most likely is similar between fetus and adult animals.

Neonatal Mineral Metabolism

Fetal survival during the birthing process may require a substantial antioxidant capacity to counter the anoxic conditions experienced, especially in the case of a prolonged dystocia.[40,41] Most trace minerals in addition to vitamins A and E serve as systemic antioxidants. During the early postnatal period, almost all essential nutrients are adequately provided for by milk consumption. However, most trace minerals, namely Cu, Fe, Zn, and Se, are insufficiently provided by milk consumption alone (see **Table 2**), thus requiring additional sources to meet daily needs. These sources may include dry feed consumption or mobilization of tissue reserves, if available, or both. Fetal hepatic nutrient reserves play a critical role in maintaining adequate trace mineral concentrations to support daily nutrient requirements in the milk-fed postnatal animal. Hepatic mineral reserves are augmented by consumption of colostrum, a moderately concentrated source of most essential trace minerals.

Nutrient concentrating ability of the fetal liver can only partially compensate for maternal nutrient deficiencies in helping to maintain normal function in postnatal life. Beef calves born to cows fed Se-adequate, Se-marginal, or Se-deficient diets showed significant differences in their Se status, measured as Se-dependent glutathione peroxidase activity, at birth and 8 weeks postnatally.[42] Calves born to cows fed the Se-deficient diet had the lowest glutathione peroxidase activity at birth and 8 weeks and showed a 36% decline in enzyme activity compared with only a 17% decline in calves from Se-adequate dams.[42] This study also showed a significant dietary effect on colostral Se concentration but no significant effect on milk Se concentration as the dietary Se source was an inorganic form. Extrapolating from this study, sufficiency of fetal hepatic mineral reserves might explain differences in time frame and severity of specific nutrient deficiency disease occurrence during early postnatal life. Recognizing most trace minerals are involved not only in metabolic activities but also in immune function, one could surmise inadequate fetal mineral resources to support postnatal life may induce a compromised immune response and greater susceptibility to disease.

MINERAL DIAGNOSTIC EVALUATION

Understanding the role of mineral nutrition in animal health has prompted a need for accurate assessment and interpretation of mineral status relative to disease risk or diagnosis. Newer analytical technologies allow rapid measurement of multiple mineral concentrations in blood or tissue samples. Diagnostic interpretation of adult animal blood or hepatic mineral concentrations is reasonably defined.[16,43,44] Diagnostic criteria for fetal and neonatal hepatic mineral concentrations are available but being further developed for ruminant species.[39] More controlled feeding trial research studies are needed to specifically determine adequate hepatic mineral concentrations in ruminant species fetal and neonatal samples.

In attempting to determine mineral status, one needs to consider what question is being asked. First, if one is interested in determining the cause-effect relationship between deficiency of a mineral and specific pathologic lesion, then one needs to look at the physiologic or biochemical role of the mineral relative to its biochemical function. More often the issue of consequence is determining the nutritive status of the animal. The former question is answered by measuring some aspect of the biochemical function pool, whereas the latter is answered by measuring the storage pool mineral content. Unfortunately, serum or whole blood is the specimen of choice due to the ease of sample collection. Interpretation of this pool can be difficult in many circumstances due to dynamic circumstances of nutrient flux through this pool and the fact that serum trace mineral concentrations are influenced by the presence of an inflammatory response associated with any disease process.[17,29,45] Interpretation of blood mineral concentrations can be augmented by collecting multiple samples although this adds to diagnostic costs.[17,29,46] As a result, a liver biopsy specimen is the preferred sample to determine trace mineral nutritive status of the animal. With application of new mass spectroscopy methods, less-invasive liver biopsies collecting approximately 20-30 mg of wet tissue can provide a sufficient sample size.[47] Liver samples can be obtained from any portion of the liver as no evidence of significant mineral concentration variation within the liver has been documented.[44,48]

Given described differences between fetal and maternal mineral metabolism and understanding neonatal mineral metabolism is a gradual progression from fetal to adult metabolic patterns, it seems obvious adult-based wet weight diagnostic criteria cannot be used for either fetal or neonatal evaluation. Some diagnostic laboratories have recognized these differences and have established age-based criteria.[17,39,49] A confounding issue here is the application of dry weight determination. Although dry weight concentrations are appropriate for comparisons due to changing tissue moisture content with advancing age, dry matter determination may vary by laboratory method and sample handling. **Fig. 2** presents bovine fetal liver dry matter ratio over gestational age for two abattoir studies and a collection of diagnostic laboratory abortion submissions. The relationship between fetal age and liver dry matter content is linear and similar across these data, but there is much variation among diagnostic samples most likely due to sample handling, autolysis, and other issues altering moisture content. Ludwick and colleagues[50] suggested hepatic potassium content could reflect liver moisture in bovine samples although this mineral is not routinely

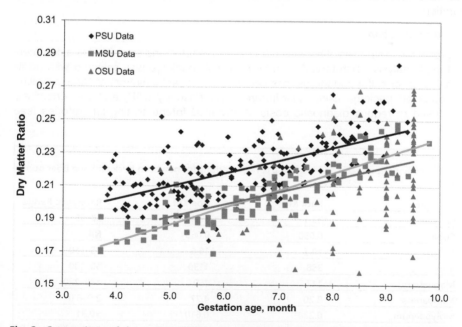

Fig. 2. Comparison of dry matter (DM) ratios for bovine fetuses (dairy and beef) based on estimated gestational age for different study populations. Both PSU and MSU studies were abattoirs samples, whereas OSU study was diagnostic lab abortion samples. Modeled equations based on fetal age were: PSU, $y = 0.0078x + 0.171$ $r^2 = 0.43$; MSU, $y = 0.0105x + 0.1346$ $r^2 = 0.79$; OSU, $y = 0.0077x + 0.153$ $r^2 = 0.13$.

measured. Care should be taken in preventing desiccation of liver samples during collection, storage, and shipment. Samples can be frozen and submitted frozen to the laboratory to minimize moisture changes in transit.

CASE STUDY OF GOAT KID LOSSES

A Boer goat breeder submitted two stillborn kids to the Penn State Animal Diagnostic Laboratory for necropsy. History indicated a high rate of stillborn and weak kids, resulting in loss of 29 kids during the current kidding season. Eight does had also been lost during kidding, and a lower pregnancy efficiency occurred during the breeding season. Herd size was approximately 60 breeding does. A similar kid loss event occurred 3 years ago and was suspected to been caused by *Chlamydophila* infection.

Diagnostic Testing and Assessment

The two submitted kids (buck and doe) had slight to moderate amount of milk curd in the abomasum indicating they had nursed briefly. Necropsy findings were unremarkable in the buck kid, and the doe kid had diffuse subacute interstitial pneumonia with a positive culture for *Mannheimia haemolytica* as well as some contaminate bacteria. Chlamydia was not identified in either kid. No congenital malformations externally or internally were identified. Liver mineral and vitamin E concentrations were determined (**Table 3**). Fecal samples were collected from the doe herd with fecal egg counts ranging from 100 to 3,700 eggs per gram determined. Necropsy findings focused on the low liver copper and vitamin E concentrations in the two kids, and the case was referred to the Penn State field investigation unit to address herd nutrition.

Dietary Evaluation

Representative samples of harvested hay were collected and submitted to a commercial feed analysis laboratory. A standard analysis package was selected with additional tests for sulfur and Mo as these are two significant inhibitors of Cu availability. A combined package using near-infrared spectroscopy (NIR) and wet chemistry was used to reduce diagnostic costs. Accredited forage testing laboratories (see

Table 3
Reported hepatic mineral and vitamin E concentrations for newborn buck and doe Boer goat kids

Nutrient	Buck Kid	Doe Kid	Reference Range
Calcium	85.1	77.4	30–65
Cobalt	0.050	0.063	NA
Copper	10.5	16.6	25–150
Iron	388	1130	50–130
Magnesium	117	150	130–220
Manganese	8.20	4.77	2.0–6.0
Molybdenum	0.234	0.610	>0.31
Selenium	0.293	0.308	0.25–1.20
Zinc	14.0	35.4	25–120
Vitamin E	<0.5	1.8	3.3–6.6

All values are presented as μg/g on a wet weight basis.

Table 4
Determined nutrient composition of harvested hay and guaranteed analysis of a commercial goat mineral product for a Boer goat herd experiencing doe and kid death losses

Parameter	Units	Grass Hay #1, 1st Cutting 2013	Grass Hay #2, 2nd Cutting 2012	Commercial Goat Mineral[a]
Dry matter (DM)	%	87.6	89.3	99
Crude protein (CP)	%DM	10.4	14.9	
Soluble protein	%CP	27.6	17.3	
Rumen degradable protein	%CP	63.8	58.6	
Total digestible nutrients	%DM	58.6	59.1	
Acid detergent fiber	%DM	39.3	38.4	
Neutral detergent fiber	%DM	65.0	59.8	
Ash	%DM	6.67	9.39	
Nonfiber carbohydrates	%DM	17.1	14.5	
Calcium	%DM	0.39	0.85	15.5–18.5
Phosphorus	%DM	0.28	0.28	8.0
Magnesium	%DM	0.11	0.29	1.5
Potassium	%DM	2.35	2.95	1.0
Salt	%DM			18.5–22.0
Sodium	%DM	0.005	0.008	7.0–8.4
Sulfur	%DM	0.21	0.24	NL
Iron	ppm	56	98	NL
Manganese	ppm	33	79	NL
Zinc	ppm	26	51	7500
Copper	ppm	6	9	1450–1850
Molybdenum	ppm	2.25	3.09	NL
Selenium	ppm			26

Abbreviation: NL, not listed.
[a] Information from guaranteed analysis of product.

www.foragetesting.org) have excellent NIR calibrations for basic forage nutrient analyses and recognize minerals cannot be accurately determined by NIR, thus the use of wet chemistry. A guaranteed analysis on the feed label from the commercial free-choice goat mineral product provided a basic nutrient analysis. A custom grain mix was made on farm and consisted of corn, roasted soybeans, and molasses and fed at a rate of 1 lb/doe/day.

The nutrient composition of the two hay forages and the commercial free-choice goat mineral are presented in **Table 4**. First-cut hay from the current year was a mature grass forage of reasonable quality. Second-cut hay from the previous year was a better-quality less-mature grass forage. Of interest relative to the case situation was the measured Cu and Mo content of the forage. Forage Cu is typical for the geographic area; however, the Mo content is higher than expected. The sulfur content was within expected values. The interaction between Cu, Mo, and sulfur in ruminants is well defined and results in reduced dietary Cu availability.[51,52] A dietary Cu:Mo ratio below 4:1 will reduce Cu availability and lead to marginal to clinical Cu deficiency. These forages had Cu:Mo ratios of 2.7:1 and 2.9:1, both potentially inducing Cu deficiency. The commercial mineral had high Cu content between 1450 and 1850 mg/kg (parts per million).

Table 5
Dietary evaluation of Boer goat herd experiencing reproductive issues and high postnatal kid losses

Early-Mid Gestation	As Fed (kg)	DMI (kg)	TDN (kg/d)	NDF (kg/d)	CP @20% (g/d)	Ca (g/day)	P (g/day)	Salt (g/day)	Cu (mg/day)	Mo (mg/day)
Corn	0.123	0.11	0.10	0.01	10.82	0.02	0.31	0.03	0.24	0.00
Roasted soybean	0.082	0.08	0.06	0.01	30.50	0.31	0.54	0.08	1.71	0.00
Molasses cane	0.023	0.02	0.01	0.00	0.99	0.17	0.02	0.09	1.12	0.00
Orchard grass 1st cut	0.000	0.00	0.00	0.00	0.00	0.00	0.00	0.00	0.00	0.00
Orchard grass 2nd cut	1.250	1.12	0.66	0.67	166.32	9.49	3.13	0.00	10.05	3.45
Mineral	0.000	0.00	0.00	0.00	0.00	0.00	0.00	0.00	0.00	0.00
Total nutrients supplied	1.48	1.32	0.83	0.69	208.64	9.99	4.00	0.20	13.12	3.45
Nutrients required		1.25	0.66	0.50	124	5.7	3.2	2.53	25.0	0.00
Difference		0.07	0.17	0.19	84.64	4.29	0.80	(2.33)	(11.88)	3.45
Dietary concentration		89.2%	63%	52%	15.8%	0.76%	0.30%	0.01%	9.96	2.62
%BW or ratios		2.6%		1.4%		2.50			3.8:1	

Diet consisted of a second cutting grass hay with a grain mix comprising corn, roasted soybeans, and molasses.

Abbreviations: BW, body weight; Ca, calcium; CP, crude protein; Cu, copper; DMI, dry matter intake; NDF, neutral detergent fiber; P, phosphorus; TDN, total digestible nutrients; Mo, molybdenum.

These are summated or calculated differences for the nutrients presented as follows: Total nutrients supplied = sum of nutrient for all ingredients of the diet; Nutrients required = NRC recommended requirement for the described animal; Difference = the subtraction of required amounts from supplied amounts; Dietary concentration = calculated concentration of the nutrient in the diet; %BW or ratios = nutrient presented as intake amount as a percent of body weight or the calculated ratio betwen the two nutrients.

A summary of a spreadsheet assessment of the mid-gestation diet for this farm is shown in **Table 5**. Using the better-quality forage and 0.5 lb of the grain mix, the diet is appropriately balanced for the macronutrients of concern. Dietary Cu is deficient, and the Cu:Mo ratio is below 4:1, supportive of a Cu deficiency situation. This represents the fed diet without the mineral. In questioning the owner, it seems there was a strong association of herd health and reproduction problems with mineral expenditures (low mineral usage was consistent with poor herd performance).

Final Diagnosis and Recommendations

Although clinical signs consistent with Cu deficiency were not observed, diagnostic findings and dietary evaluation supported a diagnosis of Cu deficiency or subclinical deficiency. Adding one-half ounce (14 grams) of the commercial mineral provided approximately 20 mg of Cu, which balanced the diet to the Cu requirement with a more appropriate Cu:Mo ratio (9.6:1). The recommended dietary ratio of Cu:Mo for goats is between 6:1 and 10:1. A recommendation was to incorporate 0.5 ounce of the mineral into the daily grain mix and to increase this to 0.75 ounce for does in late pregnancy. A follow-up communication with the owner indicated much improved doe reproductive efficiency and greatly reduced kid losses.

CLINICS CARE POINTS

- Ensuring sufficient trace mineral supplementation during pregnancy is essential to support fetal development and for survival and health in the early postnatal nursing period.

- Collecting fresh liver samples from abortion, stillbirth, or neonatal deaths and submitting for mineral analysis is suggested as an ongoing monitoring method of the herd or flock's transition mineral program.

- Dietary analysis is a critical component to evaluating mineral programs. In ruminant trace mineral concerns, one needs to evaluate potential inhibitors such as sulfur, iron, and molybdenum in the diet and water.

- Blood analysis can be used to assess trace mineral status, but interpretation is best made when collecting multiple samples.

DISCLOSURES

Grant funding was received from Pennsylvania Department of Agriculture, United States, American Dairy Goat Association, United States, Zoetis, United States.

REFERENCES

1. Suttle NF. Mineral nutrition of livestock. 4th edition. Oxfordshire, UK: CABI International; 2010.
2. Goff JP. Invited review: Mineral absorption mechanisms, mineral interactions that affect acid-base and antioxidant status, and diet considerations to improve mineral status. J Dairy Sci 2018;101:2763–813.
3. Hostetler CE, Kincaid RL, Mirando MA. The role of essential trace elements in embryonic and fetal development in livestock. Vet J 2003;166:125–39.
4. Graham TW, Thurmond MC, Mohr FC, et al. Relationships between maternal and fetal liver copper, iron, manganese, and zinc concentrations and fetal development in California Holstein dairy cows. J Vet Diagn Invest 1994;6:77–87.

5. Van Saun R. Hepatic mineral concentrations and health status in bovine fetuses. 14th International Congress of Production Diseases in Farm Animals 2010;167–8.

6. Orr JP, Blakley BR. Investigation of the selenium status of aborted calves with cardiac failure and myocardial necrosis. J Vet Diagn Invest 1997;9:172–9.

7. Van Loo H, Pascottini OB, Ribbens S, et al. Retrospective study of factors associated with bovine infectious abortion and perinatal mortality. Prev Vet Med 2021; 191:105366.

8. Wolf-Jackel GA, Hansen MS, Larsen G, et al. Diagnostic studies of abortion in Danish cattle 2015-2017. Acta Vet Scand 2020;62:1.

9. Anderson ML, Blanchard PC, Barr BC, et al. A survey of causes of bovine abortion occurring in the San Joaquin Valley, California. J Vet Diagn Invest 1990;2: 283–7.

10. Berglund B, Steinbock L, Elvander M. Causes of stillbirth and time of death in Swedish Holstein calves examined post mortem. Acta Vet Scand 2003;44:1–10.

11. Toombs RE, Wikse SE, Kasari TR. The incidence, causes, and financial impact of perinatal mortality in North American beef herds. Vet Clin North Am Food Anim Pract 1994;10:137–46.

12. Waldner CL. Cow attributes, herd management and environmental factors associated with the risk of calf death at or within 1h of birth and the risk of dystocia in cow–calf herds in Western Canada. Livest Sci 2014;163:126–39.

13. Waldner CL, Blakley B. Evaluating micronutrient concentrations in liver samples from abortions, stillbirths, and neonatal and postnatal losses in beef calves. J Vet Diagn Invest 2014;26:376–89.

14. Van Saun RJ. Paying attention to the small things: trace minerals and vitamins impact pregnancy wastage. Livestock 2018;23:180–7.

15. Suttle N. Problems in the diagnosis and anticipation of trace element deficiencies in grazing livestock. Vet Rec 1986;119:148–52.

16. Radke SL, Ensley SM, Hansen SL. Inductively coupled plasma mass spectrometry determination of hepatic copper, manganese, selenium, and zinc concentrations in relation to sample amount and storage duration. J Vet Diagn Invest 2020; 32:103–7.

17. Herdt TH, Hoff B. The use of blood analysis to evaluate trace mineral status in ruminant livestock. Vet Clin North Am Food Anim Pract 2011;27:255–83, vii.

18. House WA, Bell AW. Mineral accretion in the fetus and adnexa during late gestation in Holstein cows. J Dairy Sci 1993;76:2999–3010.

19. House WA, Bell AW. Sulfur and selenium accretion in the gravid uterus during late gestation in Holstein cows. J Dairy Sci 1994;77:1860–9.

20. National Research Council (NRC). Nutrient requirements of small ruminants: sheep, goats, cervids, and new world camelids. Washington, DC: The National Academies Press; 2007.

21. National Academies of Sciences, Engineering, and Medicine (NASEM). Nutrient requirements of dairy cattle: eighth revised edition. Washington, DC: The National Academies Press; 2021.

22. National Academies of Sciences, Engineering, and Medicine (NASEM). Nutrient requirements of beef cattle: eighth revised edition. 8th ed. Washington, DC: The National Academies Press; 2016.

23. Battaglia F, Meschia G. Principal substrates of fetal metabolism. Physiol Rev 1978;58:499–527.

24. Bell AW, Ehrhardt RA. Regulation of placental nutrient transport and implications for fetal growth. Nutr Res Rev 2002;15:211–30.

25. Abdelrahman M, Kincaid R. Deposition of copper, manganese, zinc, and selenium in bovine fetal tissue at different stages of gestation. J Dairy Sci 1993;76: 3588–93.
26. Gooneratne S, Christensen D. A survey of maternal and fetal tissue zinc, iron, manganese and selenium concentrations in bovine. Can J Anim Sci 1989;69: 151–9.
27. Hidiroglou M. Trace elements in the fetal and neonate ruminant: a review. Can Vet J 1980;21:328.
28. Hidiroglou M, Knipfel J. Maternal-fetal relationships of copper, manganese, and sulfur in ruminants. A review. J Dairy Sci 1981;64:1637–47.
29. Ensley S. Evaluating mineral status in ruminant livestock. Vet Clin North Am Food Anim Pract 2020;36:525–46.
30. Fry R, Spears J, Lloyd K, et al. Effect of dietary copper and breed on gene products involved in copper acquisition, distribution, and use in Angus and Simmental cows and fetuses. J Anim Sci 2013;91:861–71.
31. Goff JP, Stabel JR. Decreased plasma retinol, α-tocopherol, and zinc concentration during the periparturient period: effect of milk fever. J Dairy Sci 1990;73: 3195–9.
32. Goff JP, Kimura K, Horst RL. Effect of mastectomy on milk fever, energy, and vitamins A, E, and β-carotene status at parturition. J Dairy Sci 2002;85:1427–36.
33. Van Saun RJ, Herdt TH, Stowe HD. Maternal and fetal selenium concentrations and their interrelationships in dairy cattle. J Nutr 1989;119:1128–37.
34. Abuelo A, Mann S, Contreras GA. Metabolic factors at the crossroads of periparturient immunity and inflammation. Vet Clin North Am Food Anim Pract 2023;39: 203–18.
35. Anas M, Diniz WJS, Menezes ACB, et al. Maternal mineral nutrition regulates fetal genomic programming in cattle: a review. Metabolites 2023;13:593.
36. Gooneratne S, Christensen D. A survey of maternal copper status and fetal tissue copper concentrations in Saskatchewan bovine. Can J Anim Sci 1989;69:141–50.
37. Van Saun RJ, Herdt TH, Braselton WE. Hepatic trace-mineral concentrations in the bovine fetus and neonate. 34th Annual Conference of American Association of Bovine Practitioners 2001;205.
38. Van Saun RJ. Interrelationships between maternal and fetal mineral status: a new perspective. American Association of Bovine Practitioners Conference Proceedings 2019;378-378.
39. Van Saun R. Mineral and Vitamin deficiencies in aborted and stillborn calves. In: Szenci O, Mee J, Bleul U, et al, editors. Bovine prenatal, perinatal and neonatal medicine. First ed. Budapest, Hungary: Hungarian Association for Buiatrics; 2021. p. 246–60.
40. Mutinati M, Piccinno M, Roncetti M, et al. Oxidative stress during pregnancy in the sheep. Reprod Domest Anim 2013;48:353–7.
41. Mutinati M, Pantaleo M, Roncetti M, et al. Oxidative stress in neonatology: a review. Reprod Domest Anim 2014;49:7–16.
42. Koller L, Whitbeck G, South P. Transplacental transfer and colostral concentrations of selenium in beef cattle. Am J Vet Res 1984;45:2507–10.
43. Stowe HD, Braselton WE, Kaneene JB, et al. Multielement assays of bovine tissue specimens by inductively coupled argon plasma emission spectroscopy. Am J Vet Res 1958;46:561–5.
44. Braselton WE, Stuart KJ, Mullaney TP, et al. Biopsy mineral analysis by inductively coupled plasma—atomic emission spectroscopy with ultrasonic nebulization. J Vet Diagn Invest 1997;9:395–400.

45. Kincaid R. Assessment of trace mineral status of ruminants: a review. Proceedings of the American Society of Animal Science 1999;77(1):1–10.
46. Herdt TH, Rumbeiha W, Braselton WE. The use of blood analyses to evaluate mineral status in livestock. Vet Clin North Am Food Anim Pract 2000;16:423–44.
47. Herdt TH. Liver Biopsy Procedure in Cattle. 2021. Available at: https://cvm.msu.edu/vdl/laboratory-sections/nutrition/mineral-and-vitamin-testing-sample-collection-and-handling/liver-biopsy-procedure-in-cattle. Accessed March 20, 2023.
48. Abdelrahim A, Wensing T, Schotman A. Distribution of iron and copper in the liver and spleen of veal calves in relation to the concentration of iron in the diet. Res Vet Sci 1986;40:209–11.
49. Puschner B, Choi Y-K, Tegzes JH, et al. Influence of age, sex, and production class on liver zinc concentration in calves. J Vet Diagn Invest 2004;16:278–82.
50. Ludwick TP, Poppenga RH, Green PG, et al. The correlation of potassium content and moisture in bovine liver samples analyzed for trace mineral concentrations. J Vet Diagn Invest 2008;20:314–20.
51. Smith B, Wright H. Copper: Molybdenum interaction: Effect of dietary molybdenum on the binding of copper to plasma proteins in sheep. J Comp Pathol 1975;85:299–305.
52. Suttle N. The interactions between copper, molybdenum, and sulphur in ruminant nutrition. Annu Rev Nutr 1991;11:121–40.

Evaluation of Trace Mineral Sources

Jerry W. Spears, PhD*

KEYWORDS

- Trace mineral sources • Injectable trace minerals • Trace mineral boluses • Copper
- Selenium • Zinc

KEY POINTS

- Trace mineral supplementation is often needed to correct or prevent trace mineral deficiencies.
- Trace minerals can be added to the diet, provided in free-choice supplement or administered strategically as a long-acting rumen bolus or in an injectable form.
- Several trace mineral sources are commercially available for dietary supplementation, including inorganic forms, numerous organic sources, and hydroxychloride forms, and these sources can differ in their bioavailability.
- Replacing all or a portion of inorganic trace minerals with organic sources has resulted in variable responses in milk production, growth, reproduction, and claw integrity.

INTRODUCTION

One or more trace minerals are required for virtually all biochemical processes in the body. Several trace minerals function as essential cofactors for enzymes involved in metabolic processes. Other trace minerals are involved in normal functioning of vitamins or hormones. A severe deficiency of an essential trace mineral generally results in clinical signs of deficiency that can only be corrected by supplementation of the deficient mineral. Severe trace mineral deficiencies in ruminants in the United States are rare today, but marginal trace mineral deficiencies are more likely. Marginal trace mineral deficiencies can reduce growth, milk production, reproduction, or health in ruminants showing few, if any, clinical signs of deficiency.

Forages or other feedstuffs consumed by ruminants provide an important source of trace minerals. Little is known regarding bioavailability of trace minerals present naturally in feeds. However, one should not assume that trace minerals in feeds are totally unavailable; this is clear from studies where trace mineral supplementation has not affected performance or health.[1,2]

Department of Animal Science, North Carolina State University, Raleigh, NC 27695-7621, USA
* 135 Rock Bridge Road, Gallatin, TN 37066.
E-mail address: Jerry_Spears@ncsu.edu

Vet Clin Food Anim 39 (2023) 413–424
https://doi.org/10.1016/j.cvfa.2023.05.002

In many situations ruminant diets are deficient or at least marginally deficient in one or more trace minerals, requiring trace mineral supplementation for optimal performance. Many supplemental sources and methods of supplementation are available. Trace mineral source can affect bioavailability of the mineral for essential functions.[3] Source of trace minerals supplemented also may affect rumen fermentation, and limited research suggests that trace mineral source affects microflora in the lower gut. This article reviews trace mineral sources and methods of delivery.

INORGANIC TRACE MINERAL SOURCES

The cheapest sources of supplemental trace minerals are inorganic sources. Inorganic forms include sulfate, oxide, and carbonate sources. Sulfate sources of trace minerals are water soluble, whereas oxide and carbonate sources have a very low solubility in water. Oxide and carbonate trace mineral sources are at least partially soluble under acidic conditions. Different feed-grade sources of a particular mineral (sulfate, oxide, and so forth) can also differ in purity and other factors that affect bioavailability of the mineral.

Copper sulfate is the most bioavailable inorganic copper source. Copper carbonate was only 41% as effective in increasing liver copper concentrations as copper sulfate in copper-deficient heifers.[4] Feed-grade copper oxide is essentially unavailable in cattle. Supplementation of copper oxide to copper-deficient calves did not increase plasma copper relative to noncopper supplemented calves.[5] Copper oxide is relatively insoluble even under acidic conditions and apparently passes through the abomasum before the copper can be solubilized.

Zinc oxide is much more soluble under acidic conditions than copper oxide. When incubated in 0.12 N HCl for 1 hour, 2 feed-grade zinc oxide sources were 99% soluble.[6] Studies in lambs suggest that zinc sulfate and zinc oxide are similar in bioavailability.[3] Two feed-grade sources of manganese oxide were 70% and 53% as bioavailable as reagent-grade manganese sulfate in lambs.[3]

Bioavailability of selenium from selenite and selenate is similar in cattle and sheep.[3] Absorption of inorganic selenium is much lower in ruminants than in nonruminants. The lower selenium absorption in ruminants is believed to be due to reduction of inorganic selenium to insoluble forms, such as selenide or elemental selenium, by ruminal microorganisms.[3] Iodate, iodide, and ethylenediamine dihydroiodide (EDDI) are highly bioavailable sources of iodine. Calcium iodate and EDDI are generally preferred in mineral mixes because iodide sources are less stable and losses can occur due to heat, moisture, light, and exposure to other minerals. Cobalt carbonate and cobalt sulfate are the major sources of cobalt used in ruminant diets and free-choice mineral supplements. Bioavailability of cobalt seems to be similar for both sources.[7] This suggest that, despite its low solubility in water, rumen bacteria that synthesis vitamin B_{12} are capable of obtaining cobalt from cobalt carbonate.

ORGANIC TRACE MINERALS
Selenium and Chromium

All supplemental selenium and chromium sources must be approved by the US Food and Drug Administration (FDA) before being used in animal diets. Two organic selenium sources (selenium yeast and hydroxy-selenomethionine) have been approved by FDA and can be added to ruminant diets at up to 0.30 mg Se/kg dry matter. Selenomethionine is the predominant form of selenium that occurs naturally in feedstuffs and organic selenium sources. Organic selenium is taken up by ruminal microorganisms to a greater extent than inorganic selenium.[8,9] The greater uptake of organic selenium by microorganisms may increase selenium bioavailability by reducing the amount of dietary selenium reduced to insoluble forms in the rumen. Selenomethionine and selenium yeast were approximately twice as bioavailable as selenite, based on erythrocyte glutathione peroxidase (selenium-containing enzyme) activity, when supplemented to selenium-deficient heifers.[10] Glutathione peroxidase activity has generally not been greatly affected by selenium source when selenium has been provided at adequate levels.[11,12] However, organic selenium supplementation results in greater concentrations of selenium in blood, milk, liver, and muscle than inorganic selenium, especially when added to diets in quantities greater than requirements.[13,14] Selenomethionine can be used to synthesize selenium requiring enzymes or be incorporated into nonspecific proteins in place of methionine. The greater selenium concentration in blood, milk, and tissues in ruminants fed organic versus inorganic selenium is primarily due to selenomethionine incorporation into general proteins, when selenium is supplemented to diets adequate in selenium.[3]

Chromium functions by enhancing insulin sensitivity. Since 2009 chromium propionate has been permitted for addition to cattle diets. Chromium propionate is currently the only chromium source approved by FDA for supplementation to cattle diets and can be added at concentrations up to 0.5 mg Cr/kg dry matter. Approval of chromium propionate in cattle was largely based on utility and human food safety studies. The utility study indicated that chromium propionate supplementation increased insulin sensitivity, following intravenous glucose infusion.[15] The human food safety study demonstrated that chromium propionate supplementation did not increase chromium concentrations in meat and milk to levels that might cause a human health concern.[16]

Chromium propionate supplementation at 0.25 mg Cr/kg or 0.45 mg Cr/kg diet has increased gain and hot carcass weights in some studies[17,18] but not in others.[19] In calves purchased at action barns and transported to a feedlot, chromium propionate supplementation at 0.30 mg Cr/kg diet improved gain and feed efficiency and reduced the number of calves treated at least once for respiratory symptoms during a 56-day receiving period.[20]

In peak lactation dairy cows, chromium propionate supplementation increased dry matter intake and tended to improve energy-corrected milk yield.[21] Providing chromium propionate to dairy cows during the transition period seems to produce carryover effects on milk production after removal of supplemental chromium at 28 or 35 days post partum. Cows that received chromium propionate during the transition period tended to produce more milk through 84 or 90 days of lactation than cows not receiving chromium propionate.[22,23]

Zinc, Copper, and Manganese

Numerous sources of organic zinc, copper, and manganese are available commercially. Organic sources of these metals include those classified as metal proteinates, amino acid complexes, amino acid chelates, metal methionine hydroxy analogue chelates, and polysaccharide complexes. Many of the classified organic sources are produced by more than one supplier. Organic metals are covalently bonded to one or more ligand, using amino acids or polysaccharides. If the metal chelate or complex is stable in at least a portion of the digestive tract, the metal should be somewhat protected from forming complexes with dietary components that inhibit absorption and thus be more available for absorption.

It is generally believed that organic trace minerals are more bioavailable than inorganic sources. However, there is limited evidence to support the concept that organic trace minerals are considerably better absorbed than good quality sulfate forms. Some research with organic forms of copper suggests higher absorption than from copper sulfate during stress[24] or in situations where dietary molybdenum and sulfur are high.[25] In contrast other studies have found no differences in bioavailability of copper from organic sources and copper sulfate.[26,27] Studies in lambs[28] and cattle[24] indicated that apparent absorption of zinc from zinc methionine and inorganic zinc oxide or zinc sulfate was similar. Plasma and tissue zinc concentrations have also been similar in ruminants fed organic or inorganic zinc when zinc has been supplemented at normal to low supplementation rates. Based on tissue manganese accumulation in lambs fed high dietary manganese, relative bioavailability of manganese from manganese methionine was 120% of that present in manganese sulfate.[29]

It is unclear how various organic trace mineral sources compare. Organic zinc sources vary in their solubility in water and also in their bioavailability based on tissue zinc concentrations in lambs fed high levels of zinc.[30] Two copper proteinate sources differed in their water solubility. However, their bioavailability was similar when supplemented at low levels to diets of copper-depleted heifers.[4] In studies that have compared organic trace mineral sources in beef cattle[31,32] or lactating dairy cows,[33] production responses (growth or milk production) have generally been similar. Interpretation of these results is difficult because cattle supplemented with inorganic trace minerals have generally performed similarly to those receiving organic sources in these studies.

Animal responses to organic trace minerals in ruminants have been highly variable. A complete review of studies evaluating organic trace minerals is beyond the scope of this article. This article selectively describes some of the responses that have been observed to replacing inorganic with organic trace mineral sources.

Organic trace minerals may improve claw integrity. Supplementation of a zinc polysaccharide complex or zinc proteinate to fattening bulls for 284 days improved claw status compared with those receiving zinc oxide or no supplemental zinc.[31] Partial replacement of sulfate trace minerals with amino acid complexes reduced the incidence of heel erosion in lactating dairy cows exhibiting a low incidence of heel erosion.[34] In dairy studies where the incidence of heel erosion was high, supplementing amino acid complexes has not reduced heel erosion incidence.[35,36] Partial replacement of sulfate trace minerals with amino acid complexes from approximately 70 days prepartum until 36 weeks post partum reduced the incidence of sole ulcers in dairy cows.[35] Lactating dairy cows supplemented with zinc glycinate had a lower fecal relative abundance of Treponema spp than those receiving zinc sulfate.[37] Bovine digital dermatitis has been associated with Treponema bacteria in dairy cows.

In a long-term study covering 2 dry periods and 2 lactations, complete or partial replacement of sulfate trace minerals with amino acid complexes increased milk production.[34] Other studies have also reported increased milk production in dairy cows fed amino acid complex forms of copper, zinc, and manganese compared with all sulfates.[38] In contrast several studies have reported similar milk production in dairy cows supplemented with organic and sulfate trace minerals.[36,39,40] Lactating dairy cows supplemented with polysaccharide complexes[33] or amino acid complexes[38] had fewer days open than cows receiving only sulfate trace minerals. In other studies, reproductive performance of lactating dairy cows has not been affected by trace mineral source.[34–36,39]

Performance of feedlot cattle fed inorganic and organic trace minerals has generally been similar.[1,31,32] In a 2-year study beef cows were offered a control (no supplemental copper, zinc, or manganese) free-choice mineral supplement or the same supplemented with copper, zinc, and manganese from either sulfate or metal proteinate sources from approximately 82 days prepartum until calves were weaned.[41] Calf weaning weights in this study were not affected by trace mineral level or source.

Control cows tended to have lower overall pregnancy rate over the 2-year study. Trace mineral source did not affect reproduction. Following weaning calves were shipped to a feedlot and remained on their same treatment throughout the growing and finishing phase.[1] Gain and carcass characteristics were not affected by trace mineral treatment. Feed efficiency was greater during the growing and finishing phase for calves supplemented with metal proteinates versus sulfates in year 1 but not in year 2 of the study. In a more recent study, Angus and Brangus cows receiving a free-choice mineral containing organic trace minerals during the last trimester of gestation and lactation produced calves with greater weaning weights than cows supplemented with sulfate forms.[42] In a 3-year study, young (3–4 years of age) Braford cows receiving organic trace minerals had greater pregnancy rates than those fed sulfate sources in 2 of the 3 years.[43] Reproduction was not affected by trace mineral source in mature cows.

Organic trace minerals may affect rumen fermentation. Digestibility of neutral detergent fiber (NDF) and acid detergent fiber (ADF) was greater in lambs supplemented with copper proteinate compared with those receiving copper sulfate.[44] Lambs supplemented with zinc methionine or zinc proteinate had greater ADF and crude protein digestibility than lambs supplemented with zinc sulfate.[45] Steers receiving zinc, copper, and manganese complexes had higher NDF and ADF digestibility than those supplemented with sulfate forms.[46] Limited research in lambs suggest that zinc provided as an amino acid complex may affect the rumen bacterial community differently than zinc sulfate.[47]

HYDROXYCHLORIDE TRACE MINERALS

Hydroxychloride trace minerals are a fairly new category of trace minerals. In contrast to sulfates where the metal is bound to sulfate via weak ionic bonds, the metals in hydroxychloride trace minerals are covalently bonded to multiple hydroxy groups. Hydroxychloride trace minerals are relatively insoluble at neutral pH but become soluble under acidic conditions typical of those in the abomasum of ruminants. Bioavailability of copper hydroxychloride relative to copper sulfate was 132% to 196% in steers fed diets high in the copper antagonists, molybdenum, and sulfur.[48] Apparent absorption and retention of zinc was higher in steers supplemented with 25 mg Zn/kg from zinc hydroxychloride compared with those receiving zinc sulfate.[49] Beef cows receiving a free-choice mineral supplement containing zinc and copper hydroxychloride had greater liver zinc and copper concentrations than cows offered a mineral containing a combination of 75% sulfates and 25% amino acid complexes of zinc and copper.[50]

The metabolism of zinc and copper hydroxychloride in the rumen differ greatly from sulfate forms. Steers dosed with sulfate trace minerals had much higher ruminal soluble zinc and copper concentrations after dosing than steers given hydroxychloride sources.[51,52] In contrast zinc and copper concentrations in ruminal solid digesta were much higher in steers dosed with hydroxychloride trace minerals. Based on their release following dialysis against a chelating agent (ethylenediaminetetraacetic acid [EDTA]), copper and zinc from hydroxychloride forms were less tightly bound to ruminal solid digesta than sulfate forms.[51,52] The greater bioavailability of hydroxychloride forms of zinc and copper may relate to their weaker binding to ruminal solid digesta. The weaker binding of copper and zinc to the solid digesta likely relates to hydroxychloride forms interacting less with antagonists in the rumen environment.

Studies have indicated that hydroxychloride and sulfate trace minerals differ in their effect on rumen fermentation. Lactating dairy cows supplemented with hydroxychloride sources of zinc, copper, and manganese had greater NDF digestibility than those receiving sulfate sources.[53] Replacing sulfate trace minerals with hydroxychloride forms also increased NDF and ADF digestibilities in steers fed a medium quality grass hay[52] or a lactating dairy type diet.[46] The improved fiber digestion in steers receiving hydroxychloride trace minerals was associated with greater total volatile fatty acid concentrations at 0, 2, and 4 hours after feeding.[46,52]

The low water solubility of hydroxychloride trace minerals may offer some advantages in free-choice supplements. In preference trials, weaned calves showed a strong preference for trace mineral–concentrated supplements containing hydroxychloride versus sulfate or organic trace mineral sources.[54] They suggested that the low preference for sulfate and organic trace mineral supplements was due to their solubility in the mouth, creating a metallic-taste aversion. Calves offered a mineral-concentrated supplement for 84 days before weaning consumed greater amounts when the supplement contained hydroxychloride sources compared with the supplement containing zinc sulfate, copper sulfate, and manganese oxide.[54] Simulated rainfall-induced leaching losses were also greater for free-choice salt-based supplements containing sulfate or organic trace mineral sources than supplements containing hydroxychloride sources.[55]

Plasma markers of oxidative stress suggested lower oxidative stress in lactating dairy cows receiving hydroxychloride trace minerals compared with those receiving sulfates.[56] Lactating dairy cows supplemented with zinc hydroxychloride had lower fecal populations of Treponema spp than cows receiving zinc sulfate.[57] As discussed previously Treponema spp have been linked to bovine digital dermatitis.

RUMEN BOLUSES

Slow-release boluses have been used to provide copper, cobalt, selenium, and iodine over a period of time. Intake of free-choice mineral supplements varies considerably among animals in a herd and also by season.[58] Administrating a rumen bolus ensures that each animal receives the same quantity of a trace mineral. Copper oxide needle boluses have been used for some time to supply supplemental copper to ruminants. Although feed-grade copper oxide powder is poorly bioavailable, copper oxide needles supply available copper when administrated orally to ruminants. Because of their size and density, copper oxide needles are retained in the gastrointestinal tract and release copper for months. Differences in copper bioavailability between copper oxide powder and needles can be explained by the much faster rate of passage of the powder compared with the needles. The length of time that copper oxide needles will provide adequate copper depends on the copper content and level of copper antagonists present in the forage. In a copper-deficient range beef herd in Northern California, a single dose of a bolus supplying 25 g of copper oxide needles was effective in increasing liver copper for up to 8 months.[59]

Strategic supplementation with glass boluses supplying copper, selenium, and cobalt was effective in increasing liver copper and blood selenium concentrations in beef cows under range conditions.[60] Administering boluses in fall and later winter reduced calving interval and increased calf weaning weights in a 4-year study.[61]

INJECTABLE TRACE MINERALS

Injectable trace minerals provide each animal with a known quantity of trace minerals that is rapidly available for biochemical functions. In ruminants deficient in one or more trace minerals present in the product, one would expect the injected mineral to be efficiently used and a rapid response in production or health. Injectable selenium, usually in combination with vitamin E, has been used for several years to increase selenium status in cattle and sheep receiving selenium-deficient forages. In dairy cows fed diets deficient in selenium, intramuscular injections before calving have reduced duration of clinical symptoms of mastitis and incidence of retained placenta.[62]

Injectable products are also available containing zinc, copper, manganese, and selenium. Zinc, copper, and manganese in these products are chelated to EDTA to reduce inflammatory reactions of the metals at the injection site. Studies in beef cattle have clearly indicated that multielement trace mineral injections increase liver copper and selenium concentrations.[63,64] Plasma manganese concentrations also were elevated for a short period of time after injection. Calf weaning weights and steer performance have generally not been affected by trace mineral injections in cattle receiving adequate trace minerals via the diet or a free-choice mineral supplement.[64–67] Beef cows injected with trace minerals 105 days before projected calving and 30 days before fixed-time artificial insemination (AI) had a greater AI pregnancy rate than cows injected with saline.[67] However, reproductive performance has not been affected by injectable trace minerals in most beef and dairy studies. Multielement injectable trace minerals reduced morbidity and improved performance in receiving cattle exhibiting a high morbidity rate (87% in controls).[68] Trace mineral injections at arrival in the feedlot have not affected morbidity in receiving cattle when morbidity rate has been low in controls (15%–32%).[69,70]

In a study conducted on 3 dairy farms in New York, treated cows were given multielement trace mineral injections at approximately 230 and 260 days of gestation and at 35 days post partum.[71] Cows injected with trace minerals had similar milk production to controls but reduced incidence of subclinical mastitis (8 vs 10.4%), endometritis (28.6 vs 34.2), and stillbirths (4.3 vs 6.1%).

SUMMARY

Several trace mineral sources, including inorganic, numerous organic, and hydroxychloride sources, are available for dietary supplementation or inclusion in a free-choice supplement. Inorganic forms of copper and manganese differ in their bioavailability. Although research results have been variable, organic and hydroxychloride trace minerals are generally considered more bioavailable than inorganic sources. Research indicates that fiber digestibility is lower in ruminants fed sulfate trace minerals compared with hydroxychloride and some organic sources. Strategic administration of long-acting rumen boluses or injectable trace minerals are alternative methods of supplementation. Compared with free-choice supplements, individual dosing with rumen boluses or injectable forms ensures that each animal receives the same quantity of a trace mineral.

CLINICS CARE POINTS

- Trace mineral deficiencies can impair growth, milk production, reproduction, and/or health in ruminants.
- Inorganic, organic, and hydroxychloride trace mineral sources are available for dietary supplementation, and these forms can differ in bioavailability.
- In dairy cows and feedlot cattle trace minerals can best be supplemented in the total mixed ration.
- In cattle grazing pastures trace mineral can be provided in free-choice supplement or by strategic administration of a slow-release rumen bolus or in an injectable form.

- An injectable trace mineral provides a rapidly available source of mineral for animals deficient in a trace mineral but provides little or no benefit in ruminants with adequate trace mineral status.

DISCLOSURE

J.W. Spears has received research funding from Alltech, United States, Animax Ltd, Kemin Agri Foods North America, Micronutrients USA LLC, and Zinpro Corporation,- United States. He currently consults for Kemin and Micronutrients.

REFERENCES

1. Ahola JK, Sharpe LR, Dorton KL, et al. Effects of lifetime copper, zinc, and manganese supplementation and source on performance, mineral status, immunity, and carcass characteristics of feedlot cattle. Prof Anim Sci 2005;21:305–17.
2. Berrett CJ, Wagner JJ, Neuhold KL, et al. Comparison of National Research Council standards and industry trace mineral supplementation strategies for yearling feedlot steers. Prof Anim Sci 2015;31:237–47.
3. Spears JW. Trace mineral bioavailability in ruminants. J Nutr 2003;133:1506S–9S.
4. Ward JD, Spears JW. Bioavailability of copper proteinate and copper carbonate relative to copper sulfate in cattle. J Dairy Sci 1996;79:127–32.
5. Kegley EB, Spears JW. Bioavailability of feed-grade copper sources (oxide, sulfate, or lysine) in growing cattle. J Anim Sci 1994;72:2728–34.
6. Sandoval M, Henry PR, Littell RC, et al. Estimation of the relative bioavailability of zinc from inorganic zinc sources for sheep. Anim Feed Sci Technol 1997;66:223–35.
7. Kawashima T, Henry PR, Ammerman CB, et al. Bioavailability of cobalt sources for ruminants. 2. Estimation of the relative value of reagent grade and feed grade sources from tissue cobalt accumulation and vitamin B_{12} concentrations. Nutr Res 1997;17:957–74.
8. Mainville AM, Odongo NE, Bettger, et al. Selenium uptake by ruminal microorganisms from organic and inorganic sources in dairy cows. Can J Anim Sci 2009;89:105–10.
9. Galbraith ML, Vorachek WR, Estill CT, et al. Rumen microorganisms decrease bioavailability of inorganic selenium supplements. Biol Trace Elem Res 2016;171:338–43.
10. Pehrson B, Knutsson M, Gyllensward M. Glutathione peroxidase activity in heifers fed diets supplemented with organic and inorganic selenium compounds. Swedish J Agric Res 1989;19:53–6.
11. Ortman K, Pehrson B. Effect of selenate as a feed supplement to dairy cows in comparison to selenite and selenium yeast. J Anim Sci 1999;77:3365–70.
12. Juniper DT, Rymer C, Briens M. Bioefficacy of hydroxy-selenomethionine as a selenium supplement in pregnant dairy heifers and on the selenium status of their calves. J Dairy Sci 2019;102:7000–10.
13. Juniper DT, Phipps RH, Ramos-Morales, et al. Effect of dietary supplementation with selenium-enriched yeast or sodium selenite on selenium tissue distribution and meat quality in beef cattle. J Anim Sci 2008;86:3100–9.
14. Sun P, Wang J, Liu W, et al. Hydroxy-selenomethionine: A novel organic selenium that improves antioxidant status and selenium concentrations in milk and plasma of mid-lactation dairy cows. J Dairy Sci 2017;100:9602–10.

15. Spears JW, Whisnant CS, Huntington GB, et al. Chromium propionate enhances insulin sensitivity in growing cattle. J Dairy Sci 2012;95:2037–45.
16. Lloyd KE, Fellner V, McLeod SJ, et al. Effects of supplementing dairy cows with chromium propionate on milk and tissue chromium concentrations. J Dairy Sci 2010;93:4774–80.
17. Budde AM, Sellins K, Lloyd KE, et al. Effect of zinc source and concentration and chromium supplementation on performance and carcass characteristics in feedlot steers. J Anim Sci 2019;97:1286–95.
18. Baggerman JO, Smith ZK, Thompson AJ, et al. Chromium propionate supplementation alters animal growth performance, carcass characteristics, and skeletal muscle properties in feedlot steers. Transl Anim Sci 2020;4:1–14.
19. Edenburn BM, Kneeskern SG, Bohrer BM, et al. Effects of supplementing zinc or chromium to finishing steers fed ractopamine hydrochloride on growth performance, carcass characteristics, and meta quality. J Anim Sci 2016;94:771–9.
20. Bernhard BC, Burdick NC, Rounds W, et al. Chromium supplementation alters the performance and health of feedlot cattle during the receiving period and enhances their metabolic response to a lipopolysaccharide challenge. J Anim Sci 2012;90:3879–88.
21. Vargas-Rodriguez CF, Yuan K, Titgemeyer EC, et al. Effects of supplemental chromium propionate and rumen-protected amino acids on productivity, diet digestibility, and energy balance of peak-lactation dairy cows. J Dairy Sci 2014;97: 3815–21.
22. McNamara JP, Valdez F. Adipose tissue metabolism and production responses to calcium propionate and chromium propionate. J Dairy Sci 2005;88:2498–507.
23. Rockwell RJ, Allen MS. Chromium propionate supplementation during the prepartum period interacts with starch source fed postpartum: Production responses during the immediate postpartum and carryover periods. J Dairy Sci 2016;99: 4453–63.
24. Nockels CF, DeBonis J, Torrent J. Stress induction affects copper and zinc balance in calves fed organic and inorganic copper and zinc sources. J Anim Sci 1993;71:2539–45.
25. Hansen SL, Schlegel P, Legleiter LR, et al. Bioavailability of copper from copper glycinate in steers fed high dietary sulfur and molybdenum. J Anim Sci 2008;86: 173–9.
26. Ward JD, Spears JW, Kegley EB. Effect of copper level and source (copper lysine vs copper sulfate) on copper status, performance, and immune response in growing steers fed diets with and without supplemental molybdenum and sulfur. J Anim Sci 1993;71:2748–55.
27. Sinclair LA, Hart KJ, Johnson D, et al. Effect of inorganic or organic copper fed without or with added sulfur and molybdenum on the performance, indicators of copper status, and hepatic mRNA in dairy cows. J Dairy Sci 2013;96:4355–67.
28. Spears JW. Zinc methionine for ruminants: Relative bioavailability of zinc in lambs and effects on growth performance of growing heifers. J Anim Sci 1989;67: 835–43.
29. Henry PR, Ammerman CB, Littell RC. Relative bioavailability of manganese from a manganese-methionine complex and inorganic sources for ruminants. J Dairy Sci 1992;75:3473–8.
30. Cao J, Henry PR, Guo R, et al. Chemical characteristics and relative bioavailability of supplemental organic zinc sources for poultry and ruminants. J Anim Sci 2000;78:2039–54.

31. Kessler J, Morel I, Dufey PA, et al. Effect of organic zinc sources on performance, zinc status and carcass, meat and claw quality in fattening bulls. Livestock Prod Sci 2003;81:161–71.

32. Malcolm-Callis KJ, Duff GC, Gunter SA, et al. Effects of supplemental zinc concentration and performance, carcass characteristics, and serum values in finishing beef steers. J Anim Sci 2000;78:2801–8.

33. Chester-Jones H, Vermeire D, Brommelsiek W, et al. Effect of trace mineral source on reproduction and milk production in Holstein cows. Prof Anim Sci 2013;29:289–97.

34. Nocek JE, Socha MT, Tomlinson DJ. The effect of trace mineral fortification level and source on performance of dairy cows. J Dairy Sci 2006;89:2679–93.

35. Siciliano-Jones JL, Socha MT, Tomlinson DJ, et al. Effect of trace mineral source on lactation performance, claw integrity, and fertility in dairy cows. J Dairy Sci 2008;91:1985–95.

36. DeFrain JM, Socha MT, Tomlinson DJ, et al. Effect of complexed trace minerals on the performance of lactating dairy cows on a commercial dairy. Prof Anim Sci 2009;25:709–15.

37. Faulkner MJ, Wenner BA, Solden LM, et al. Source of supplemental dietary copper, zinc, and manganese affects fecal microbial relative abundance in lactating dairy cows. J Dairy Sci 2017;100:1037–44.

38. Ballantine HT, Socha MT, Tomlinson DJ, et al. Effects of feeding complexed zinc, manganese, copper, and cobalt to late gestation and lactating dairy cows on claw integrity, reproduction, and lactation performance. Prof Anim Sci 2002;18:211–8.

39. Hackbart KS, Ferreira RM, Dietsche AA, et al. Effect of dietary organic zinc, manganese, copper, and cobalt supplementation on milk production, follicular growth, embryo quality, and tissue mineral concentrations in dairy cows. J Anim Sci 2010;88:3856–70.

40. Mion B, Van Winters B, King K, et al. Effects of replacing inorganic salts of trace minerals with organic trace minerals in pre- and postpartum diets on feeding behavior, rumen fermentation, and performance of dairy cows. J Dairy Sci 2022;105:6693–709.

41. Ahola JK, Baker DS, Burns PD, et al. Effect of copper, zinc, and manganese supplementation and source on reproduction, mineral status, and performance in grazing beef cattle over a two-year period. J Anim Sci 2004;82:2375–83.

42. Price DM, Arellano KK, Irsik M, et al. Effects of trace mineral source during gestation and lactation in Angus and Brangus cows and subsequent calf immunoglobulin concentrations, growth and development. Prof Anim Sci 2017;33:194–204.

43. Arthington JD, Swenson CK. Effects of trace mineral source and feeding method on the productivity of grazing Braford cows. Prof Anim Sci 2004;20:155–61.

44. Dezfoulian AH, Aliarabi H, Tabatabaei MM, et al. Influence of different levels and sources of copper supplementation on performance, some blood parameters, nutrient digestibility and mineral balance in lambs. Livestock Sci 2012;147:9–19.

45. Alimohamady R, Alliarabi H, Bruckmaier R, et al. Effect of different sources of supplemental zinc on performance, nutrient digestibility, and antioxidant enzyme activities in lambs. Biol Trace Elem Res 2019;189:75–84.

46. Guimaraes O, Wagner JJ, Spears JW, et al. Trace mineral source influences digestion, ruminal fermentation, and ruminal copper, zinc, and manganese distribution in steers fed a diet suitable for lactating dairy cows. Anim 2022;16. https://doi.org/10.1016/j.animal.2022.100500.

47. Ishaq SL, Page CM, Yeoman CJ, et al. Zinc AA supplementation alters yearling ram rumen bacterial communities but zinc sulfate does not. Transl Anim Sci 2019;97:687–97.

48. Spears JW, Kegley EB, Mullis LA. Bioavailability of copper from tribasic copper chloride and copper sulfate in growing cattle. Anim Feed Sci Technol 2004; 116:1–13.

49. Shaeffer GL, Lloyd KE, Spears JW. Bioavailability of zinc hydroxychloride relative to zinc sulfate in growing cattle fed a corn-cottonseed hull-based diet. Anim Feed Sci Technol 2017;232:1–5.

50. Jalali S, Lippolis KD, Ahola JK, et al. Influence of supplemental copper, manganese, and zinc source on reproduction, mineral status, and performance in a grazing beef cow-calf herd over a 2-year period. Appl Anim Sci 2020;36:745–53.

51. Caldera E, Weigel B, Kucharczyk VN, et al. Trace mineral source influences ruminal distribution of copper and zinc and their binding strength to ruminal digesta. J Anim Sci 2019;97:1852–64.

52. Guimaraes O, Jalali S, Wagner JJ, et al. Trace mineral source impacts rumen trace mineral metabolism and fiber digestion in steers fed a medium-quality grass hay diet. J Anim Sci 2021;99. https://doi.org/10.1093/jas/skab220.

53. Faulkner MJ, Weiss WP. Effect of source of trace minerals in either forage- or by-product-based diets fed to dairy cows: Production and macronutrient digestibility. J Dairy Sci 2017;100:5358–67.

54. Caramalac LS, Netto AS, Martins PGMA, et al. Effects of hydroxychloride sources of copper, zinc, and manganese on measures of supplement intake, mineral status, and pre- and postweaning performance of beef calves. J Anim Sci 2017;95: 1739–50.

55. Arthington JD, Silveira ML, Caramalac LS, et al. Effects of varying sources of Cu, Zn, and Mn on mineral status and preferential intake of salt-based supplements by beef cows and calves and rainfall-induced metal loss. Transl Anim Sci 2021;5. https://doi.org/10.1093/tas/txab046.

56. Yasui T, Ryan CM, Gilbert RO, et al. Effects of hydroxy trace minerals on oxidative metabolism, cytological endometritis, and performance of dairy cows. J Dairy Sci 2014;97:3728–38.

57. Wenner BA, Park T, Mitchell K, et al. Effect of zinc source (zinc sulfate or zinc hydroxychloride) on relative abundance of fecal Treponema spp. in lactating dairy cows. J Dairy Sci 2022;3. https://doi.org/10.3168/jdsc.2022-0238.

58. Cockwill CL, McAllister TA, Olson ME, et al. Individual intake of mineral and molasses supplements by cows, heifers and calves. Can J Anim Sci 2000;80: 681–90.

59. Graham TW, Thurmond MC, Galey FD. Efficacy of copper oxide wire supplementation on repletion of copper stores in range beef cattle in Northern California. Agri Pract 1995;16. number 8.

60. Sprinkle JE, Cuneo SP, Frederick HM, et al. Effects of a long-acting, trace mineral, reticulorumen bolus on range cow productivity and trace mineral profiles. J Anim Sci 2006;84:1439–53.

61. Sprinkle JE, Schafer DW, Cuneo SP, et al. Effects of a long-acting trace mineral rumen bolus upon range cow productivity. Transl Anim Sci 2021;5. https://doi.org/10.1093/tas/txaa232.

62. Spears JW, Weiss WP. Role of antioxidants and trace elements in health and immunity of transition dairy cows. Vet J 2008;176:70–6.

63. Genther ON, Hansen SL. A multielement trace mineral injection improves liver copper and selenium concentrations and manganese superoxide dismutase activity in beef steers. J Anim Sci 2014;92:695–704.

64. Stokes RS, Volk MJ, Ireland FA, et al. Effect of repeated trace mineral injections on beef heifer development and reproductive performance. J Anim Sci 2018;96: 3943–54.

65. Genther-Schroeder ON, Hansen SL. Effects of a multielement trace mineral injection before transit stress on inflammatory response, growth performance, and carcass characteristics of beef steers. J Anim Sci 2015;93:1767–79.

66. Stokes RS, Ireland FA, Shike DW. Influence of repeated trace mineral injections during gestation on beef heifer and subsequent calf performance. Transl Anim Sci 2019;3:493–503.

67. Mundell LR, Jaeger JR, Waggoner JW, et al. Effects of prepartum bolus injections of trace minerals on performance of beef cows and calves grazing native range. Prof Anim Sci 2012;28:82–8.

68. Richeson JT, Kegley EB. Effect of supplemental trace minerals from injection on health and performance of highly stressed, newly received beef heifers. Prof Anim Sci 2011;27:461–6.

69. Clark JH, Olson KC, Schmidt TB, et al. Effects of respiratory disease risk and a bolus injection on growing and finishing performance by beef steers. Prof Anim Sci 2006;22:245–51.

70. Roberts SL, May ND, Brauer CL, et al. Effect of injectable trace mineral administration on health, performance, and vaccine response of newly received feedlot cattle. Prof Anim Sci 2016;32:842–8.

71. Machado VS, Bicalho MLS, Pereira RV, et al. Effect of an injectable trace mineral supplement containing selenium, copper, zinc, and manganese on the health and production of lactating Holstein cows. Vet J 2013;197:451–6.

Trace Mineral Nutrition in Confinement Dairy Cattle

Robert B. Corbett, DVM, PAS, Dipl. ACAN

KEYWORDS

• Trace minerals • Deficiency • Toxicosis • Diagnosis • Requirements

KEY POINTS

- Veterinarians may be called upon to diagnose problems with trace mineral toxicities or deficiencies but often do not have sufficient information as to feeding rates.
- Ration analysis may indicate sufficient trace mineral concentrations are being fed, however, deficiencies may be present because of high interfering mineral concentrations reducing absorption.
- Routine forage analysis often does not include all trace minerals necessary to adequately assess presence of mineral interactions that may result in trace mineral deficiency.
- Many feed companies and nutrition groups have standard trace mineral-vitamin premix formulas used regardless of geographic location and trace mineral concentrations in soil and forages.
- Diagnosis of trace mineral deficiencies or toxicoses depends upon appropriate samples collection according to the trace mineral being considered, followed by accredited laboratory analysis.

INTRODUCTION

Whenever the milk prices drop, a significant percentage of dairy owners look at their ration costs as a possible area to cut operating expenses. One of the highest cost items in the ration is the mineral, especially the trace minerals. In times of severe cash flow distress, many farms have been forced to make cutbacks in their mineral supplementation to better maintain cash flow.

Dairies that have opted to remove the trace minerals from their rations often feel that their cows have not shown any negative effects because of not having trace minerals in their diet and, for this reason, are reluctant to add these back into the diet because of the cost. It is important for the veterinarian to understand the role of these trace minerals in the health and productivity of the dairy cow so that the long-term consequences of restricting these minerals in the diet can be evaluated. Also, as the level of milk production continues to increase throughout the United States on an annual basis, it becomes more important to fine tune dairy cow rations and pay more

Dairy Health Consultation, PO Box 100, Spring City, UT 84662, USA
E-mail address: cowdoc@dairy-health.com

Vet Clin Food Anim 39 (2023) 425–438
https://doi.org/10.1016/j.cvfa.2023.06.004
0749-0720/23/© 2023 Elsevier Inc. All rights reserved.

vetfood.theclinics.com

attention to detail in providing the optimum level of nutrition to the high-production dairy cow. Trace mineral and vitamin nutrition is often overlooked as a potential way of optimizing the health and production of the lactating dairy cow. Veterinarians need to be aware of the signs of both trace mineral deficiencies and toxicoses that may occur in their client's dairies.

Trace Mineral Sources

Regional differences in soil type, climate, available forages, grains and byproducts, mineral composition of the water, and other factors all have a significant impact on the concentrations of trace minerals and vitamins that are naturally available in the ration. The only way to make sure that the trace mineral nutrition of a particular herd is adequate is to analyze the concentrations of trace minerals in blood samples and liver biopsies. The samples should be collected from healthy animals in various stages of lactation as well as dry cows and close-ups. It is very common for nutritionists and feed companies to have a "standard" trace mineral-vitamin pack that is used in all rations on the farm, or at least in all adult cow rations, regardless of the geographic area the dairy is located in. These "standard" trace mineral-vitamin premixes could be significantly problematic if the dairyman is using a nutritionist from a larger nationwide nutritional service that uses the same premix in all geographic areas. There will be many instances where more trace mineral is provided than is needed, and there can be cases where not enough is provided because of various interactions that may exist as will be discussed in the following sections. This trace mineral-vitamin package is usually the most expensive part of the ration. If analysis of the trace mineral status of the herd indicates that some trace minerals are present in the body at higher concentrations than needed, those specific trace minerals could be reduced, resulting in significant savings in ration costs.

Absorption and Utilization of Trace Minerals

Trace mineral nutrition is very complex because of the many interactions that occur between different trace minerals. Also, proper absorption of trace minerals depends on the chemical form of the mineral that is present in the feed or mineral supplement. Consequently, an analysis of the ration may indicate that sufficient concentrations of the required trace minerals are present, but the amount absorbed by the animal may not be adequate because of the previously mentioned interactions that interfere with the absorption and utilization of trace minerals. Toxicosis due to excessive concentrations of trace minerals in the ration may also be a problem. Excessive concentrations of some trace minerals may also interfere with the absorption of another. Likewise, a deficiency of one trace mineral may result in reduced absorption or metabolism of another. Some of the major factors that affect the absorption and metabolism of trace minerals will be discussed to make the veterinarian more aware of possible problems that may exist with trace mineral nutrition in his client's dairy herd. Cobalt, copper, iodine, iron, manganese, selenium, and zinc are considered to be the most important trace minerals that are essential to the health and productivity of the dairy cow.

Cobalt

Cobalt is an essential element as the active center of coenzymes called cobalamins, which includes vitamin B_{12}. Ruminants do not absorb much glucose directly from the rumen since it is utilized by rumen bacteria as an energy source. The animal must produce the majority of its glucose from other nutrients in the body, especially propionate. Vitamin B_{12} is an essential part of an enzyme that is necessary for the conversion of propionate to glucose. Animals that are cobalt deficient cannot produce sufficient concentrations of glucose and develop symptoms that result from inadequate energy concentrations such as decreased growth rate, poor appetite, decreased milk production, and poor hair coat. Vitamin B_{12} cannot be supplemented orally because it is broken down by rumen bacteria. However, there are products commercially available that contain rumen-protected B complex vitamins, including B_{12}. B_{12} is synthesized in sufficient amounts by the rumen bacteria if adequate concentrations of cobalt are present in the diet. Rumen bacteria also synthesize other analogs of B_{12} that are present in the serum and liver. These analogs of B_{12} make it difficult to receive an accurate analysis of B_{12} concentrations in serum and liver. Therefore, the concentration of B_{12} cannot be used as a method of determining whether cobalt has been supplemented in sufficient amounts in the diet.[1] However, if liver concentrations of vitamin B_{12} are less than 0.1 µg/g wet weight, it is indicative of a cobalt deficiency.[2] Cobalt is not utilized very efficiently in the rumen, and only about 3% of what is ingested is utilized for the synthesis of vitamin B_{12} by the rumen microorganisms. It is not very effective to use cobalt as a fertilizer on crop ground to try and satisfy the animal's cobalt requirement. It should be supplemented through a salt or mineral premix and incorporated into the ration.

Because B_{12} is synthesized by rumen microorganisms, younger animals with underdeveloped rumens have lower reserves of B_{12} in the liver and are therefore more sensitive to cobalt deficiency in the diet. Common signs of cobalt deficiency in young animals would include failure to grow, unthriftiness, and loss of weight.[3] In severe cases, fatty degeneration of the liver and anemia with pale mucous membranes may be observed.[4]

There is not sufficient research data available to accurately determine the recommended dietary allowance for cobalt. The National Research Council (NRC) 2021 has established an adequate intake (AI) level of cobalt to be 0.2 mg Co/kg of diet dry matter.[5]

Cobalt toxicosis is rare and usually only occurs when there has been a major error in the formulation or manufacturing of the trace mineral premix. The signs of cobalt toxicosis are similar to the signs of cobalt deficiency, such as reduced feed intake, loss of body weight, and in severe cases, anemia.[6–8] The NRC 2005 has set the maximal tolerable dietary cobalt concentration at 25 mg/kg of dietary dry matter.[8]

Copper and Molybdenum

Copper and molybdenum are closely interrelated and will be discussed together. Copper is necessary for the activity of several enzymes involved in numerous functions in the body. Clinical signs exhibited by animals that are deficient in copper include decreased growth rates, lower fertility, rough hair coat and loss of hair pigmentation, reduced feed conversion, diarrhea, and lameness. Fragile bones and osteoporosis, cardiac failure, and anemia may also occur.[4] Copper deficiency has been associated with an increased rate of retained placentas. Calves that were fed copper-deficient diets had an increased rate of retained placentas as adults even when the copper concentrations were normal in the adult ration. Copper is required for oocyte viability, and its positive effects on oocyte development are maintained through early embryogenesis.[9,10] Lower copper concentrations can have a negative effect on immune function before classical signs of copper deficiency are observed. The neutrophils from cows that are fed insufficient concentrations of copper have a reduced ability to kill pathogenic organisms, resulting in increased susceptibility to infections and increased severity of infections, including mastitis.[11] It has been suggested that the amount of copper that is required to maintain optimal immune function is higher than that required to prevent clinical signs of copper deficiency and that copper requirements increase when an animal is mounting an immune response against an infectious disease.[12]

Copper has the greatest potential for creating a toxicosis of all the required minerals in ruminant diets, since the amount of copper that can cause toxicosis is only 4- to 10-fold greater than the amount of copper required to support normal metabolism.[13] The level of copper in the liver that is considered to cause toxicosis has not been definitively determined. However, several studies have reported that copper toxicosis occurs when liver concentrations reach 300 to 350 mg Cu/kg dry weight.[14,15] Copper toxicosis may occur when administering large doses of certain dewormers, excessive concentrations of copper added to the mineral supplement, and feeding processed litter from broilers that were fed a high-copper diet. There has also been reports of copper toxicosis resulting from cows drinking foot bath solution containing copper sulfate. Copper sulfate and copper carbonate are two of the most common sources of copper in trace mineral mixes. Copper oxide is not readily available to the animal and should be avoided as a supplemental source of copper. It is important that mineral mixes containing a copper supplement be mixed thoroughly to prevent copper toxicosis.

Cattle that are fed excessive concentrations of copper will accumulate copper in the liver. When experiencing an environmental or infectious stress event, large amounts of copper may be released into the bloodstream resulting in acute signs of copper toxicosis. This results in a hemolytic crisis characterized by hemolysis, jaundice, methemoglobinemia, hemoglobinuria, generalized icterus, widespread necrosis, and often death.[16–18]

There are several substances that interfere with copper absorption. Molybdenum is one of primary concern. Molybdenum will react in the rumen with sulfide and form a complex that interferes with copper absorption and its metabolism after absorption.[19] Therefore, high concentrations of molybdenum can induce a copper deficiency. This complex between copper and molybdenum may also interfere with molybdenum metabolism as well. It is now recommended that the copper-to-molybdenum ratio be kept at greater than 6:1, to prevent the adverse effects of molybdenum on copper. Plants that are raised on soils that have an alkaline pH will have a higher uptake of molybdenum, making a molybdenum excess in the ration more likely. Molybdenum is rarely analyzed for in routine forage analysis and can vary significantly from one area to another in the same geographic region. Nutritionists and feed companies should take into consideration the molybdenum concentrations present in the forages used on their clients' dairies when formulating the copper concentrations to feed in the trace mineral premix.

The presence of high sulfur concentrations by itself can bind copper in the form of copper sulfides. Sulfur may be present in high amounts in common feeds such as dried distiller grains and canola. A water analysis should be done on each farm to determine sulfur concentrations. It is quite common to find high sulfur concentrations in the water supply, and water is often not considered when estimating the daily intake of sulfur in the diet.

The ingestion of soil can also result in the binding of copper by silicates and other anions in clay that form insoluble complexes with copper. This is more of a problem with pasture-based dairies but can still occur on occasion in confinement dairies. It is a fairly common occurrence to observe cows eating sand and dirt from dry lots or free stalls. High iron concentrations observed in a forage analysis is usually indicative of soil contamination of that forage, usually through flood irrigation. If the intake of soil reaches 10% of diet dry matter, copper absorption may be reduced by 50%.[20]

Excessive concentrations of zinc will increase the synthesis of metallothionein within the enterocytes. Metallothionein will also bind copper. However, in most conditions, zinc is not a major factor in reducing copper absorption unless the diet contains at least twice the amount that is recommended in the diet.[21]

Iron does not seem to interfere significantly with the absorption of copper from the intestine. However, it does interfere with copper uptake by the liver, resulting in signs of copper deficiency.[22] Iron does not seem to have an appreciable effect on copper metabolism until it reaches 500 mg/kg (500 ppm) of diet dry matter.[23] Like sulfur, water may contain high concentrations of iron, and water analysis should be performed to determine iron content.

It is important to keep in mind that just because the suggested level of copper is supplemented in the diet, it does not mean that copper deficiency is not possible because of the numerous substances that interfere with copper absorption and metabolism. Liver biopsies are the most reliable method to determine if adequate amount copper is being absorbed and utilized in the body. The NRC 2005 set the maximum tolerable level (MTL) of copper at 40 mg Cu/kg of diet dry matter.

Molybdenum is important in the detoxification of many of the end products of cellular metabolism. It is also thought to be involved in iron metabolism. Molybdenum is usually present at fairly high concentrations in dairy rations, so molybdenum deficiency is rare. Signs of molybdenum toxicosis include severe scours and loss of body condition. Molybdenum supplementation of normal rations is usually unnecessary.

Iodine

The thyroid gland requires iodine for the synthesis of hormones, which are involved in regulating the rate of energy metabolism. A geographic area may be low in iodine, which may result in inadequate concentrations in the ration. Also, some plants produce natural substances called goitrogens which interfere with iodine metabolism in the body. One of the first signs of iodine deficiency in the cow is when the calf is born with an enlarged thyroid gland (goiter). Calves may be born hairless, weak, or dead. The death of the fetus may occur at any stage of gestation. Even though these signs are observed in the fetus or newborn calf, the mother will often appear normal.[24] Other signs of iodine deficiency include decreased milk production, irregular heat intervals, decreased conception rate, and an increase in retained fetal membranes.

Toxicosis due to high concentrations of iodine in the feed is highly unlikely. Signs of toxicosis may occur if high concentrations of sodium iodide are injected during the treatment of foot rot or fungal diseases or if errors were made in the formulation of the trace mineral premix. The maximal tolerable level was set at 50 mg I/kg of diet dry matter (NRC 2005). Clinical signs of iodine toxicosis include excessive nasal and ocular discharge, hyperthermia, salivation, decreased milk production, coughing, and dry scaly coats.[25] Iodine is excreted in the milk. Humans are much more sensitive to iodine than ruminants, so cows that are fed excessive amounts of iodine would create a human health concern.[26] For this reason, the Food and Drug Administration (FDA) has set the maximum level of iodine supplementation in cattle from ethylenediamine dihydriodide (EDDI) at 50 mg/d. If a lactating cow consumes 25 kg of dry matter per day, this would result in a maximum concentration of 2.0 mg I/kg of dry matter, which is approximately three times the amount considered to be needed.[5] Common sources of supplemental iodine include iodized salt, calcium iodate, and EDDI. EDDI is the the most commonly used and the most readily absorbable salt to the animal.

Iron

Iron is best known for its role in the proper functioning of hemoglobin which is necessary for the transport of oxygen in the blood. Iron is also involved in respiration, energy metabolism, and in detoxifying potentially harmful metabolic end products. Iron deficiency is very seldom observed in adult cattle because of the high level of iron that is present in most of the common feedstuffs. Therefore, there is seldom a need for supplementing additional iron to the adult dairy cow. However, iron deficiency may occur in calves that are fed milk for extended periods of time since milk is low in iron. The results of one study suggest that supplementing iron at the rate of 50 mg Fe/kg diet is adequate to maintain physiologic function in growing veal calves.[27] The MTL for iron has been set at 500 mg Fe/kg of diet dry matter (NRC 2005). Excessive concentrations of iron in the ration may result in serious consequences to the animal. Iron can inhibit the utilization of copper by two different mechanisms. Iron traps sulfide in the rumen and then releases it in the abomasum where it combines with copper to form copper sulfide, which is unavailable for absorption. Iron oxide is also a copper-trapping agent, which reduces the amount of copper available to the animal. Not only does iron oxide reduce the amount of copper available to the animal, but it is not available to the animal as an iron source either. Iron oxide is red and is commonly used as a coloring agent in some feed ingredients. It should not be added to mineral supplements for the previously stated reasons. It has also been suggested that excessive concentrations of iron interfere with phosphorous absorption. Alfalfa, grass, and small grain silages may contain significant amount of soil in them at the time of harvest. The iron in this soil is not very bioavailable, but after being stored as silage, the solubility of iron increases by approximately 20 times.[28]

Manganese

Manganese is also an essential part of several enzyme systems in the body. These enzymes are involved in the formation of cartilage and bone, fat and carbohydrate metabolism, and the disposal of reactive oxygen metabolites.[29] Through these enzyme systems, manganese is involved in the growth process, proper functioning of the immune system, and reproduction. The following signs are observed in cattle suffering from manganese deficiency.

1. Bone abnormalities including enlarged joints, shortened and weak bones, and superior brachygnathism
2. Ataxia, deafness, and equilibrium problems caused by improper development of bones in the middle ear[5]
3. Degenerative changes in tissues deficient in manganese
4. Slower to exhibit estrus, more services per conception, increased early embryonic death

The fetal skeletal system is especially sensitive to manganese deficiencies and can show clinical signs of deficiency without any clinical signs in the dam.[30] The AI level of manganese for a late-gestation Holstein cow would be about 490 mg/d, which would be approximately 40 mg of the total Mn/kg of diet dry matter. A high-production lactating Holstein cow should be given supplements with approximately 27 mg Mn/kg of diet dry matter.[5]

Of all the essential trace minerals, manganese is one of the least toxic ones. High concentrations of manganese in the ration is not considered to be a problem. Higher concentrations of manganese may need to be supplemented if excess calcium and phosphorous are present in the ration since they decrease the amount of manganese absorbed. The MTL for manganese is set at 2000 mg Mn/kg of diet dry matter (NRC 2005). However, it has been shown that a manganese level of 500 mg Mn/kg of diet dry matter leads to an increase in the clinical signs of copper deficiency in animals that are fed a copper-deficient diet.[31] Manganese sulfate, manganese chloride, manganese dioxide, and manganese carbonate are the most common supplemental inorganic sources of manganese.

Selenium

One of selenium's most important roles is that it is an essential component of the enzyme glutathione peroxidase. During the normal metabolic processes that continually take place in the body, there are numerous byproducts that are generated. Some of these byproducts may be toxic to animal tissues. One group of these toxic metabolic end products are the peroxides. Glutathione peroxidase is involved in the destruction of peroxides, making it essential in preventing damage to body tissues.[32] Vitamin E is involved in preventing the formation of peroxides and thus is closely associated with selenium. Selenium is also an essential part of another enzyme that is involved in the formation of thyroid hormone which is important in the normal utilization of energy.

Selenium and vitamin E and its effects on mastitis have been studied extensively. Ohio State researchers reported that feeding 740 IU vitamin E in conjunction with selenium injection reduced clinical mastitis by 37% during the first 3 months after calving.[33] Numerous studies since then have confirmed this relationship between selenium, vitamin E, and the immune response.

The minimum and maximum limits on selenium in the feed are fairly narrow compared to most of the other trace minerals. There are many geographic areas in the United States that are selenium deficient. In these areas, selenium supplementation is absolutely necessary to optimize the herd health and productivity of the dairy herd. The most common signs of selenium deficiency are[34]

1. Erratic or silent heat periods
2. Poor fertilization
3. Delayed conception
4. Infertility
5. Abortions
6. Birth of premature, weak, or dead calves
7. White muscle disease in calves
8. Increased rate of retained placentas
9. Uterine infections
10. Cystic ovaries

Some areas of the United States contain certain plants called accumulators, which take up and store selenium. This creates a problem with excess intake of selenium and results in signs of toxicosis. The syndrome of selenium toxicosis is often called alkali disease or blind staggers. These animals are characterized by a loss of hair, sloughing of hoofs, lameness, anemia, excessive salivation, grinding of the teeth, blindness, paralysis, and death.

There is not much room for error in maximizing herd productivity through selenium supplementation. The amount of selenium that can be added in the feed legally is stipulated by the FDA at 0.3 mg/kg of diet dry matter. Most nutritionists formulate the supplemented selenium at this level. However, there are certain areas in the United States (eg, North and South Dakota) where selenium concentrations in the soil are significantly higher. Forages grown in these areas should be analyzed for selenium. The forage selenium content should be entered into the nutrition formulation program and the trace mineral premix adjusted to account for the concentrations of selenium in the forages.

It has become a common practice to inject selenium and vitamin E combinations into closeup dry cows 2 to 3 weeks before calving to decrease the number of retained placentas and uterine infections. These selenium-vitamin E combinations often do not contain sufficient concentrations of vitamin E to maximize the immune response. In most cases, selenium should already be supplemented in the diet in sufficient concentrations to satisfy the requirements. Vitamin E can be administered at the time of calving and result in an improvement in the immune response, which may also decrease the number of new mastitis infections during the early part of lactation.

Zinc

Zinc is one of the most widely used trace minerals in the body. It is essential for the proper function of more than 200 enzymes including superoxide dismutase. It is involved in almost every major metabolic function in the body including carbohydrate metabolism, growth and repair of tissues, sexual development, reproduction, the immune system, gene regulation, hormonal regulation, neurotransmission, and apoptosis.[35] Changes in zinc concentrations within immune cells are thought to be a major regulatory mechanism that may affect the entire immune system.[36]

Zinc deficiency is observed most commonly in calves which exhibit a decrease in dry matter intake and growth rate. Testicular development may also be affected. Calves that are fed milk can absorb about 50% of the zinc in the diet. However, that amount was reduced by about 50% when soybean protein was added to the diet, likely because of the phytic acid.[37] However, phytic acid does not seem to interfere with zinc absorption in functioning ruminants. Cows on zinc-deficient diets exhibit a scaly skin around the muzzle (especially the nostrils), neck, udder, and legs, along with weakness of the hoof horn. Because of its importance in the normal functioning of the immune system, animals that are marginally low on zinc may show an increase in mastitis, somatic cell count, and other infectious diseases.[38]

Iron, copper, and sulfur may all reduce zinc absorption. However, most practical diets will not contain high-enough concentrations of these minerals to cause a zinc deficiency. If sulfur concentrations above 0.5% of diet dry matter are present, they may reduce the amount of zinc absorption.[5] The total dietary requirement for zinc ranges from 1160 to 1735 mg/d depending on milk production and dry matter intake. A 700-kg dry cow after 270 days of gestation requires 325 mg of Zn/day (NRC 2021).

Cattle can tolerate high concentrations of zinc without exhibiting signs of toxicosis. Cows fed high concentrations of zinc that induce signs of toxicosis usually show anemia, depressed growth, joint stiffness, hemorrhages into the joints, bone resorption, depraved appetite, and in severe cases, death.[39] Feed intake, copper status, and milk production are often reduced. The MTL for cattle is set at 500 mg Zn/kg of diet dry matter. Zinc sulfate is probably the most common source of supplemental zinc. Zinc carbonate and zinc oxide are also used.

Chelated Trace Minerals

It has already been previously mentioned that there are numerous interactions between minerals that may decrease the availability of certain minerals to the animal. Most of these interactions occur in the upper gastrointestinal (GI) tract. The trace mineral cation separates or dissociates from its anion, for example, the copper separates from the sulfate and is free to react with other ions in the upper GI tract. When the mineral reaches the higher pH of the lower GI tract, it can bind to several minerals, nutrients, and nonnutritive components of the digesta, such as fiber, that render it insoluble. These insoluble complexes are excreted and therefore unavailable to the animal. Trace minerals such as zinc, copper, and manganese are also available in a chelated form. The mineral is bound to an organic molecule that results in a stable complex which prevents the mineral from separating from the organic molecule in the upper GI tract. This protects the mineral from interactions with other minerals and antagonists, thus preventing the loss of essential trace minerals in the upper GI tract. These trace minerals can then be delivered to the area of the small intestine where they can be absorbed and transported into the bloodstream. Chelated trace minerals are often referred to as organic trace minerals (OTM). The organic molecule is basically a delivery system that protects the trace mineral until it reaches the appropriate site in the small intestine where it can be absorbed and then utilized in the body.

Utilizing OTM in the ration allows the nutritionist to reduce the total amount of trace mineral that is supplemented in the ration and assures a better absorption and utilization of the supplemented minerals in the body. Some of the chelates utilize an essential amino acid such as methionine or a methionine hydroxy analog which can also be utilized to satisfy some of the methionine requirement in the ration. Chelated trace minerals are more expensive but are utilized by most nutritionists as a means of ensuring adequate absorption and utilization of the supplemented trace minerals to satisfy the requirements of the animal. A reasonable goal would be to supply one-third of the trace mineral requirement of zinc, copper, and manganese with a high-quality chelated trace mineral. This should be enough to ensure the absorption of enough trace mineral to prevent a deficiency if there were interactions with other trace minerals that were blocking the absorption of the inorganic trace minerals that were being supplemented.

Selenium is also available in an organic form as selenium yeast. It has been shown that 0.75 mg/day of selenium in a selenium yeast product maintained approximately the same selenium concentrations in whole blood and milk as 3 mg/d of selenium from sodium selenite.[40] Compared to controls, feeding 300 mg/kg dry matter per day of a selenium yeast product increased 4% fat-corrected milk and altered the rumen fermentation pattern from acetate to propionate production.[41]

Trace Mineral Packages and National Research Council Requirements

Even though there are established requirements published by the NRC, it is a commonly accepted practice to include higher amounts of certain trace minerals in the ration because of the interactions previously described that block or interfere with the absorption of specific trace minerals.

It is not common for the dairymen or veterinarian to know the level of trace minerals that are being fed to a specific herd, or what percentage of the trace mineral is being provided by the more-readily-available chelated organic sources. The trace mineral-vitamin package is often proprietary for that specific nutritionist or company. Since the formula is often not included in the ration, it is difficult for the dairyman to compare bids from different nutritionists or mineral formulators when they are using different trace mineral-vitamin premixes. Since this part of the ration is often the most expensive one, a difference of $20-$100 per ton of complete mineral mix is common, and the main difference may be what is contained in the trace mineral-vitamin premix. A cheaper mineral may not contain organic chelated trace minerals, may contain a smaller percentage of chelates, or may contain lower total concentrations of the trace minerals in the formula. In general, you pay for what you get. It would be next to impossible to compare bids from different mineral companies without knowing the formula for the trace mineral premix. It is important to know if the animals are receiving the required concentrations of trace minerals and if chelated organic minerals are in the mineral premix formula.

The rumen microorganisms also have a requirement for trace minerals. The trace mineral package should contain some of the inorganic trace minerals that can be utilized in the rumen by the microorganisms to maximize rumen efficiency. Unfortunately, the amount that is required by rumen bacteria is currently unknown, but most nutritionists feel that the requirement is minor in relation to that required for absorption in the small intestine for use in the body.

Other Factors Affecting Trace Mineral Requirements

The trace mineral requirements may vary depending on the breed of dairy cow in question. Animals that are undergoing stress, especially stimulation of the immune response due to infection, have an increased demand for trace minerals, especially copper and zinc. Stressed animals often experience a decrease in feed intake, which in turn decreases the daily intake of trace minerals. Trace mineral deficiencies have also been shown to have an effect on daily dry matter intake. Therefore, optimizing the trace mineral supplementation may have a positive effect on the immune response and the daily feed intake of stressed animals.

As previously mentioned, there are numerous interactions between minerals that affect the absorption and utilization of trace minerals in the body. Do not overlook the fact that the water supply may also contain significant concentrations minerals, especially sulfates (rotten egg smell), that can interfere with the absorption and utilization of trace minerals. The only way to make sure that the dairy herd is being supplemented with the appropriate amounts of the essential trace minerals to optimize herd productivity is to collect the necessary samples for trace mineral analysis. It is advisable to have the water, forages, grains, and byproducts tested for trace mineral concentrations, especially when making a significant change in the ration.

Analyzing Trace Mineral Status

The trace mineral status in most dairy herds is unknown. Most dairy herds receive a proprietary standardized trace mineral-vitamin package from their feed supplier or nutritionist. This package is assumed to adequately fulfill all the trace mineral requirements of the animals on that farm. However, unless there is a health issue on a specific farm that is considered to be the result of a trace mineral deficiency or toxicosis, assessment of the trace mineral status on that farm is rarely performed. It is advisable for the assessment of trace mineral status to become a more routine procedure for two main reasons.

1. There may be an existing problem with either a trace mineral deficiency or toxicosis that is not resulting in significant clinical signs, or the health issue, such as low reproductive performance, is not being associated with a trace mineral deficiency.
2. If specific trace minerals are found to be present in the body at concentrations that are considered to be in the high range or slightly above, an adjustment in the trace mineral premix can be made that could result in a significant decrease in the overall cost of the ration per head per day. If the level of a trace mineral is considered to be marginally low or below, the mineral premix formula can be adjusted to compensate for it.

Blood Analysis

Blood analysis for trace minerals is not the method of choice in most cases. In the case of copper, a low level in the blood may suggest an issue with copper deficiency but is not diagnostic. A normal copper concentration in the blood does not rule out a copper deficiency since the copper concentrations in the liver may be reduced to try and maintain adequate copper concentrations in the blood. Hemolysis in blood samples creates a major issue with the accuracy of the results for many of the trace minerals. For example, iron is present within the red blood cell at approximately 100× the normal level in serum, zinc about 5×, and selenium about 1.5× to 2× (Hall J, personal communication, 2023).

Liver Biopsies

Samples from liver biopsies are the preferred choice when analyzing for trace mineral status. Liver biopsies are a relatively simple and safe procedure that can be performed on the farm. There are several excellent videos that can be accessed on YouTube that describe the liver biopsy procedure in detail. The liver biopsy may be analyzed on a wet basis or a dry basis. The veterinary diagnostic laboratory of choice should be contacted to obtain the information as to how they prefer the samples to be prepared and shipped to their lab.

Samples should be obtained from animals representative of different stages of lactation, such as far off dry cow, closeup dry cow, early lactation, and late lactation. The same would be true if assessing the trace mineral status of calves and replacement heifers. Liver samples may be collected from animals that recently died as long as they did not have a chronic illness before death which may have resulted in a depletion of trace mineral concentrations.

It is important to understand that the trace mineral concentrations in late-term fetuses, neonates, and young animals differ significantly from those of the adult animal. **Table 1** was developed by Dr. Jeffrey Hall while at Utah State University as the director

Table 1
Suggested reference range for hepatic bovine mineral concentrations (µg/g or ppm) in adult cattle and late term fetus and neonates

| Mineral | Adult Cattle | | Late Term Fetal/ Neonatal | Comments |
	Wet Weight	Dry Weight	Wet Weight	
Calcium	30–200	100–700	30–200	
Cobalt	0.020–0.200	0.067–0.667	0.010–0.100	Pre-colostrum; Post Colostrum same as adults
Chromium	0.040–3.800	0.13–12.67	0.040–3.800	
Copper	25–100	83–350	65–150	Gradual shift to adult range by 3–4 mo of age
Iron	45–300	150–1100	55–550	Gradual shift to adult range by 1–2 mo of age
Potassium	1400–4000	4667–13333	1400–4000	
Magnesium	100–250	333–875	100–250	
Manganese	2.0–6.0	6.67–20	0.9–4.5	Gradual shift to adult range by 4–5 mo of age
Molybdenum	0.10–1.40	0.33–5.0	0.10–1.40	
Sodium	600–3500	2000–11667	600–3500	
Phosphorus	2000–4500	6667–15000	2000–4500	
Lead	<0.50	<1.67	<0.50	
Selenium	0.25–0.50	0.83–2.0	0.35–0.75	Gradual shift to adult range by 3–4 mo of age
Zinc	25–100	88–350	35–125	Gradual shift to adult range by 3–4 mo of age

Data from the Utah Veterinary Diagnostic Laboratory 2019.

of the Veterinary Toxicology Laboratory that illustrates normal concentrations of trace minerals in the liver of adult bovines on both a wet and dry basis, as well as in neonates on a wet basis.

If a trace mineral excess or deficiency is present on analysis and an adjustment in the trace mineral premix is made, the veterinarian should wait about 60 days before taking new liver biopsies to assess the effect of the change on liver concentrations of that specific mineral.

SUMMARY

Feeding a standardized trace mineral premix often results in trace mineral concentrations in the liver that are in the high normal range or even slightly above. This is an opportunity for the dairyman to reduce feed costs by lowering the concentrations of these specific minerals in the premix. Most of the problems resulting from trace mineral deficiency or toxicosis are not exhibited by obvious clinical signs. Optimizing trace mineral nutrition can have a positive effect on reproductive efficiency, the immune system, milk production, abortion rate, oxidative stress, feed efficiency, and calf health, just to name a few. Routine assessment of the trace mineral status of dairy animals is rarely done. This is an important service that dairy cattle veterinarians can do that may provide important information to the dairyman, which may have a significant effect on the overall health and productivity of the dairy herd.

CLINICS CARE POINTS

- In most cases, veterinarians do not have access to the amounts of trace minerals being fed to a specific herd.
- Deficiencies or toxicities of trace minerals may be present without clinical signs.
- Accurate diagnosis of a trace mineral toxicosis or deficiency depends on collection of appropriate samples and subsequent analysis by a reputable veterinary diagnostic laboratory.
- Assessment of trace mineral status in a herd should include liver biopsies from a representative group of animals at least on an annual basis and 60 days after any changes are made in the trace mineral formula.

DISCLOSURE

The author declares no commercial or financial conflicts to disclose.

REFERENCES

1. Halpin CG, Harris DJ, Caple IW, et al. Contribution of cobalamin analogues to plasma vitamin B_{12} concentrations in cattle. Res Vet Sci 1984;37:249–51.
2. Smith RM. In: Mertz W, editor. In trace elements in human health and disease. San Diego, CA: Academic Press; 1987.
3. Smith RM. In: Odell B, Sunde R, editors. In handbook of essential trace mineral elements. New York: Marcel Dekker; 1997.
4. Underwood EJ. The mineral nutrition of livestock. 2nd edition. Slough, UK: Commonwealth Agricultural Bureaux; 1981.

5. National Academies of Sciences, Engineering, and Medicine. Nutrient requirements of dairy cattle. 8th Revised Edition. Washington DC: The National Academies Press; 2021. p. 134.
6. Ely RE, Dunn KM, Huffman CF. Cobalt toxicosis in calves resulting from high oral administration. J Anim Sci 1948;7:239–43.
7. Keener HA, Percival GP, Marrow KS. Cobalt tolerance in young dairy cattle. J Dairy Sci 1949;32:527.
8. NRC. Mineral tolerance of animals. Washington DC: The National Academies Press; 2005.
9. Gao G, Yi J, Zhang M, et al. Effects of iron and copper in culture medium on bovine oocyte maturation, preimplantation embryo development, and apoptosis of blastocysts invitro. J Reprod Dev 2007;53(4):777–84.
10. Picco SJ, Rosa DE, Anchordoquy JP, et al. Effects of copper sulphate concentrations during in vitro maturation of bovine oocytes. Theriogenology 2012;77:373–81.
11. Scaletti RW, Trammell DS, Smith BA, et al. Role of dietary copper in enhancing resistance to Escherichia coli mastitis. J Dairy Sci 2003;86:1240–9.
12. Suttle NF. Residual effects of Mycobacterium avium infection on the susceptibility of sheep to copper toxicosis and the efficacy of conservative treatment with tetrathiomolybdate. Vet Rec 2012;171:246.
13. Goff JP. Invited Review: Mineral absorption mechanisms, mineral interactions that affect acid-base and antioxidant status, and diet considerations to improve mineral status. J Dairy Sci 2018;101:2763–813.
14. Auza NJ, Olson WG, Murphy MJ, et al. Diagnosis and treatment of copper toxicosis in ruminants. J Am Vet Med Assoc 1999;214:1624–8.
15. Grace ND, Knowles S. Taking action to reduce the risk of copper toxicosis in cattle. Vet Rec 2015;177:490–1.
16. Steffen DJ, Carlson MP, Casper HH. Copper toxicosis in suckling beef calves associated with improper administration of copper oxide boluses. J Vet Diagn Invest 1997;9:443–6.
17. Underwood EJ, Suttle NF. The mineral nutrition of livestock. 3rd edition. Wallingford, UK: CABI Publishing; 1999.
18. Johnston H, Beasley L, MacPherson. Copper toxicosis in a New Zealand dairy herd. Irish Vet J 2014;67:20.
19. Suttle NF, McLauchlan M. Predicting the effects of dietary molybdenum and sulphur on the availability of copper to ruminants. Proc Nutr Soc 1976;35:22A–3A.
20. Suttle NF. Effects of age and weaning on the apparent availability of dietary copper to young lambs. J Agric Sci 1975;84:255–61.
21. Miller WJ, Amos HE, Gentry RP, et al. Long term feeding of high zinc sulfate diets to lactating and gestating dairy cows. J Dairy Sci 1989;72:1499–508.
22. Ha JH, Doguer C, Collins JF. Consumption of a high iron diet disrupts homeostatic regulation of intestinal copper absorption in adolescent mice. Am J Physiol Gastrointest Liver Physiol 2017;313:G353–60.
23. Phillippo M, Humphries WR, Garthwaite PH. The effect of dietary molybdenum and iron on copper status and growth in cattle. J Agric Sci Camb 1987;109:315–20.
24. Hemken RW. Iodine. J Dairy Sci 1970;53:1138–43.
25. Paulikova I, Kovac G, Bires J, et al. Iodine toxicosis in ruminants. Vet Med Czech 2002;47:343–50.
26. Hetzel B, Welby M. In: O'Dell BL, Sunde RA, editors. Handbook of nutritionally essential mineral elements. New York: Marcel Dekker; 1997. p. 557–81.

27. Lindt F, Blum JW. Growth performance, haematological traits, meat variables, and effects of treadmill and transport stress in veal calves supplied with different amounts of iron. Zentralbl Veterinarmed A 1994;41:333–42.
28. Hansen SL, Spears JW. Bioaccessibility of iron from soil is increased by silage fermentation. J Dairy Sci 2009;92:2896–905.
29. Miller JK, Madsen FC. Trace minerals. Large dairy herd management. Champain, IL: American Dairy Science Association; 1992. p. 289.
30. Hansen SL, Spears JW, Lloyd KE, et al. Feeding a low manganese diet to heifers during gestation impairs fetal growth and development. J Dairy Sci 2006;89: 4305–11.
31. Hansen SL, Ashwell MS, Legleiter LR, et al. The addition of high manganese to a copper-deficient diet further depresses copper status and growth of cattle. Br J Nutr 2009;101:1068–78.
32. Van Soest PJ. Nutritional Ecology of the Ruminant. 2nd Ed. Ithaca, NY: Cornell University Press; 1994. p. 129.
33. Smith KL, Harrison JH, Hancock DD, et al. *J Dairy Sci*, 67, 1984, Ensminger Publishing Company; Clovis, CA, 1293.
34. Miller JK, Madsen FC. Trace minerals. Large dairy herd management. Champain, IL: American Dairy Science Association; 1992. p. 290.
35. Ensminger ME, Olentine CG. Feeds and Nutrition. 1978; p 109.
36. Haase H, Rink L. Functional Significance of zinc-related signaling pathways in immune cells. Annu Rev Nutr 2009;29:133–52.
37. Miller WJ, Martin YG, Gentry RP, et al. 65zn and stable zinc absorption, excretion and tissue concentrations as affected by type of diet and level of zinc in normal calves. J Nutr 1968;94:391–401.
38. Cope CM, Mackenzie AM, Wilde D, et al. Effects of level and form of dietary zinc on dairy cow performance and health. J Dairy Sci 2009;92:2128–35.
39. Ensminger ME, Olentine CG. Feeds and Nutrition. Clovis, CA: Ensminger Publishing Company; 1978. p. 110.
40. Ortman K, Pehrson B. Selenite and selenium yeast as feed supplements for dairy cows. Zentralbl Veterinarmed A Aug 1997;44(6):373–80.
41. Wang C, Liu Q, Yang WZ, et al. Effects of selenium yeast on rumen fermentation, lactation performance and feed digestibilities in lactating dairy cows. Liv Sci 2009;126:239–44.

Pasture Minerals for Dairy Cattle

Ian J. Lean, BVSc, DVSc, PhD, MANZCVS[a,b,*],
Helen M. Golder, BAgSc (Hons), PhD[a,b]

KEYWORDS

- Minerals • Pastures • Forage • Crops • Micromineral • Trace elements

KEY POINTS

- Mineral requirements for cattle do not differ with production system.
- Risks of deficiency or toxicosis reflect species of plants and even cultivars present on a farm, but also reflect soils, fertilizer and effluent application, and stage of growth of the plant.
- Building an understanding of the mineral concentrations from a farm requires testing of representative samples from the farm as book or computer values are only guides.
- Temperate grasses (ryegrasses, bromes, fescues), legumes (clovers, alfalfa), and even tropical grasses contain higher concentrations of many minerals than maize silage.

 Video content accompanies this article at http://www.vetfood.theclinics.com.

DEFINITIONS
Forage

Herbage used to feed cattle and usually refers to a specific species of plant.

Sward

Is a term used to refer to the whole pasture, whether a monoculture or mixed species.

C3 Grass

Are plants that utilize the C3 carbon fixation pathway to convert CO2 into an organic compound in the photosynthesis.

C4 Grass

Utilize phosphoenolpyruvate to convert CO2 into an organic compound in photosynthesis and reduce evaporative loss of water. This is an adaptation to hotter climates.

[a] Scibus, PO Box 660, Camden, New South Wales 2570, Australia; [b] Dairy Science Group, School of Life and Environmental Sciences, Faculty of Science, The University of Sydney, PO Box 660, Camden, New South Wales, Australia
* Corresponding author.
E-mail address: ianl@scibus.com.au

Vet Clin Food Anim 39 (2023) 439–458
https://doi.org/10.1016/j.cvfa.2023.05.003

Growth Point

The point near the lower stem from which new leaves are pushed up.

INTRODUCTION

There are no differences in mineral requirements for cattle if these are pasture fed or in confined feeding. Requirements reflect the stage of life and production of milk and milk solids (eg,[1,2]). The major differences in mineral nutrition of cattle from the production system used [pasture or total mixed ration (TMR)] relate to the physical and chemical composition of the forage, amount of forage in the diet, and understanding the variation that occurs among regions and farms, in terms of the mineral content of the forage.

Mineral deficiencies in soils, and consequently forages have been well described across the world.[3–7] There are areas that have been characterized that are deficient in calcium, cobalt, copper, iodine, phosphorus, sodium, selenium, and zinc. Less frequently deficiencies in magnesium and manganese have been identified. Many of these deficient areas have been mapped across geographical regions of the world and often strongly relate to the soils present and the geology of the regions. Notwithstanding this, total soil mineral content is not always a good predictor of plant mineral content. Kao, and colleagues[8] provide a detailed description of the factors influencing uptake of soil minerals into the plant. There is a long history of awareness of mineral-deficient areas and the development of modern agriculture has been very much aided by the identification and the management of these deficiencies.

Excessive intakes of Fe, Mo, and K can result from forages with high concentrations of these minerals. Concentrations in these forages often reflect high soil concentrations of these minerals. Further, some regions and areas within region have the potential for toxicosis, in particular with Se. However, heavy metal toxicosis resulting from ingestion of pastures high in mineral content has been noted too, especially in association with industrial pollution from mining.

The mineral deficiencies or toxicoses in forages that occur, influence forage that is purchased by confined dairies or by herds that primarily graze. The key difference in risk between the TMR and grazing systems lies in the greater proportion of diet that is supplied as forage in grazing systems. The process of preserving forage, as a silage or hay, reduces the energy and protein density of a forage, sometimes as a strategic decision to increase the yield of forage in the harvest (cut) or as a result of nutrient loss in the process of cutting, storing, and feeding out the forage. Consequently, pasture-based diets can have a higher forage content to provide a similar estimated metabolizable or net energy density to TMR, hence greater exposure to the variation in mineral content of the forage.

Another difference is in the greater proportion of forage being provided as maize in many TMR-fed herds. Maize is a C4 grass that has a much lower mineral content of macro-minerals and trace minerals when mature as silage compared to grasses such as ryegrass. Further, herds, whether TMR- or pasture-fed will be more exposed to risk with greater reliance on a single site for growing feed. Lastly, but of interest is the exposure of cattle to soil ingestion with grazing pasture.

Box

The most important trace elements in practice are Co, Cu, Fe, I, Mn, Mo, Se, and Zn.

The emphasis of this article is to examine the factors that lead to best evaluating the risks for deficiency or toxicity in pasture-based herds from pastures and grazed crops. Many of the reference articles on factors influencing the mineral composition of pasture and on the mineral content are older reflecting very active research and substantial interest in the 1960's to late 1980's.

This article does not address samples taken from the cattle to determine sufficiency; that information can be found elsewhere.[9,10] However, it is important to consider that whichever samples are used e.g. blood or liver, the estimations obtained are only a guide to adequacy as essential minerals have many different functions in the animal. There are rate-limiting metabolic pathways that may well be influenced by different availabilities of minerals. There are also interactions among disease and disorder stressors, other minerals and vitamins, energy, protein and fat nutrition, other environmental factors, and genetics that will all determine the function and adequacy of intake of a particular mineral in the animal. In many cases, a production, health, or fertility response to treatment may provide the most definitive evaluation of deficiency, but such responses may be difficult to detect for more subtle deficiency states. In the field, many of these responses are confounded by changes in the pasture and environment.

UNDERSTANDING THE SOURCES OF RISK
Characterizing the Sward

The initial step in characterizing the sward is to determine the botanical composition of the sward. Pastures can be a near monoculture especially if seasonally established. Annual, Westerwold, and Italian ryegrasses (*Lolium multiflorum*), fescues (*Festuca arundinacea*), oats (*Avena sativa*), Triticale (*x Triticosecale*), Barley (*Hordeum vulgare*), and wheat (*Triticum aestivum*) are examples of this and are C3 plants (**Figs. 1–4**). While perennial plantings of ryegrass (*Lolium perenne*) approach a monoculture, frequently these are mixed swards with clovers (*Trifolium spp.*), often being co-planted. There is an increasing trend to planting ryegrass with perennial herbs such as plantain (*Plantago lanceolata L.*), chicory (*Chicorium intybus L.*) and forage brassicas (*Brassica spp.*) in some regions (**Figs. 5 and 6**).

Box

Plants with 3 Carbon (C3) metabolism tend to be more digestible than those with a four-carbon metabolism.

There are many other options for temperate crops and pastures[11,12] and some of these are noted below including bromes (*Bromus willdenowii*), and timothy (*Phleum pratense*). However, the tropical grasses that include Bermuda (*Cynodon dactylon*),

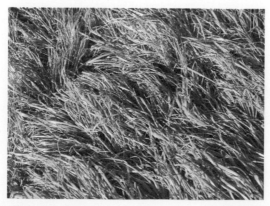

Fig. 1. Lush tetraploid Italian ryegrass.

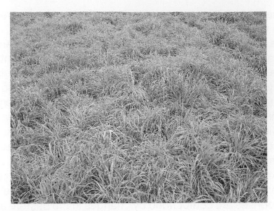

Fig. 2. Perennial ryegrass.

kikuyu (*Cenchrus clandestinum* previously, *Pennisetum clandestinum*: **Fig. 7**) and paspalum (*Paspalum dilitatum*) are important sources of grazing in regions including the South-eastern USA, Northern Australia, South America (eg, Colombia), and South Africa. Summer crop options commonly used include sorghum (*Sorghum bicolor*) which is often hybridized with sudangrass, millets, grazing maize (*Zea mays*), soyabean (*Glycine max*), cowpeas (*Vigna unguiculata*), and lablab (*Lablab purpureus*).

Uptake of minerals varies with plant species, soil composition, fertilizer application, the stage of development of the plant and can be influenced by contamination with soil and the availability of minerals in soil may differ among plants.[13] Further, the distribution of minerals varies within the plant. For example, leaf from perennial ryegrass and *Trifolium pratense* (red clover) contained higher mineral concentrations of Ca, P, Mg, Cu, Mo, and Zn than stem,[14] but this effect may not apply to Cu in lablab.[5] Senescent pastures can have lower mineral concentrations as leaching and maturity influence concentrations. However, for Cu, Fe, Mn, and Zn concentrations can be higher in dead material than in growing tissue.[6] Hence, there is considerable variation in the mineral content of ingested forage. This variation is reflected in the wide range of minerals in plants in all substantial surveys.

The information presented in **Table 1** can only be a guideline to mineral concentrations of the forages tested at one particular laboratory (Dairy One Forage Laboratory,

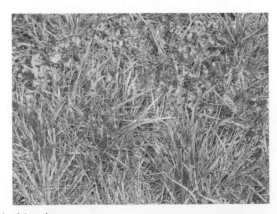

Fig. 3. Fescue and white clover.

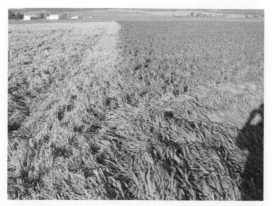

Fig. 4. Crop of oats.

Ithaca, NY), and while these provide valuable insights into the mean, range, and standard deviation, readers are cautioned that samples are those submitted to a laboratory for analysis and may not be representative, nor collected in an ideal manner; some pastures were heavily represented (eg Bahia *Paspalum notatum*). The data were provided by Dairy One based on submissions from years 2013 to 2022 and were sorted according to the evident identity of submissions and included data from North and South America, Australia, New Zealand and South Africa. Where no clear forage species was defined, samples were coded according to the submission codes reflecting mixed pastures legume dominant, mixed swards pasture dominant, and pasture swards. Outlying observations were removed from the data before the final analysis. The corn silage data were obtained from the Dairy One Library on line. The key benefit of providing this information is to explore expected concentrations regarding the risk of health disorders.

For example, many of the pastures in **Table 1** are marginal to deficient in Cu and with the high Mo, S, and Fe content present within the ranges reported, conditioned Cu deficiency can be expected to be prevalent. Similarly, dietary cation-anion difference (*DCAD*) concentrations have a range which indicates that cows fed a substantial proportion of their diet on these pastures will be at risk of hypocalcemia. In particular,

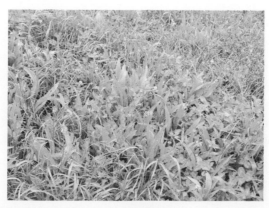

Fig. 5. Plantain, ryegrass, and clover mixed pasture.

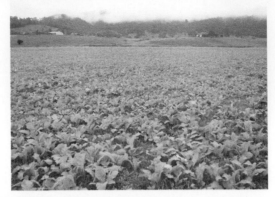

Fig. 6. Brassica and ryegrass mixed pasture.

the propensity for kikuyu pastures to accumulate K is evident with a mean DCAD of > 400 meq/kg.

Similarly, feed-banks associated with nutritional software or NASEM[1] are useful guides to likely mineral content and availability, however, testing of forage using wet chemistry methods from a particular farm can be used to build up a picture of the likely mineral risks on a farm. While concentrations of some minerals eg Ca, P, K, Mg, S, and Na can have adequate estimation using near-infra-red reflectance spectroscopy, most trace elements of nutritional significance are not well predicted[15–17] and require wet chemistry determination.

Box

The risk of mineral deficiency or excess on a farm is better understood by regular sampling of feeds to determine mineral status. For trace minerals, wet chemistry testing is required.

Selecting representative samples

Cattle have the capacity to select a much different sward to that on offer (Video 1).[18] In experimental studies oesophageal fistulated cattle have been used to obtain forage samples to understand the impact of selective grazing.

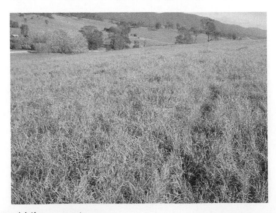

Fig. 7. Newly planted kikuyu pasture.

Table 1
Mineral concentrations (mean, minimum, maximum, and SD) of various forages tested at DairyOne Forage Testing Laboratory (Ithaca, NY)

Mineral	Alfalfa (Lucerne)	Clover	Pasture (Legume Dominant)	Ryegrass	Kikuyu	Fescue	Bahia	Bermuda	Pasture (Grass Dominant)	Pasture (Grass)	Corn/Maize (Silage)
N	437	17	134	46	178	41	579	23	3050	7549	221002
Ca											
Mean	1.1	1.12	0.98	0.5	0.39	0.45	0.44	0.6	0.46	0.51	0.23
Min	0.5	0.79	0.32	0.2	0.2	0.24	0.18	0.3	0.08	0.07	0.15
Max	2	1.5	1.93	1.5	0.76	0.82	1.18	1	1.58	1.9	0.32
SD	0.3	0.2	0.36	0.3	0.09	0.14	0.13	0.2	0.17	0.2	0.09
P											
Mean	0.4	0.45	0.37	0.4	0.49	0.35	0.19	0.3	0.33	0.22	0.24
Min	0.3	0.18	0.04	0.2	0.21	0.19	0.04	0.1	0.03	0.02	0.2
Max	0.6	0.71	0.66	0.6	0.67	0.53	0.57	0.4	0.88	0.94	0.27
SD	0.1	0.12	0.1	0.1	0.06	0.09	0.09	0.1	0.15	0.15	0.04
Mg											
Mean	0.5	0.37	0.28	0.2	0.45	0.28	0.3	0.2	0.24	0.18	0.16
Min	0.2	0.21	0.15	0.2	0.25	0.15	0.1	0.1	0.03	0.03	0.13
Max	0.8	0.76	0.49	0.4	0.71	0.5	0.62	0.4	0.83	0.99	0.2
SD	0.1	0.14	0.07	0.1	0.11	0.08	0.08	0.1	0.11	0.1	0.04
K											
Mean	2.5	2.39	2.58	3.7	4.31	2.42	0.96	1.5	2.14	1.43	1.08
Min	1	1.53	0.19	1.6	1.87	0.99	0.06	0.4	0.13	0.06	0.81
Max	5	3.15	4.6	5.6	6.04	4.27	2.71	2.8	6.47	5.75	1.35
SD	0.8	0.51	0.67	1	0.63	0.79	0.47	0.6	1.04	0.96	0.27

(continued on next page)

Table 1 (continued)

Mineral		Afalfa (Lucerne)	Clover	Pasture (Legume Dominant)	Ryegrass	Kikuyu	Fescue	Bahia	Bermuda	Pasture (Grass Dominant)	Pasture (Grass)	Corn/Maize (Silage)
Na	Mean	0.3	0.35	0.06	0.3	0.11	0.04	0.02	0.1	0.08	0.03	0.04
	Min	0	0.01	0	0	0.02	0	0	0	0	0	0
	Max	0.7	0.85	0.64	0.8	0.39	0.32	0.58	0.3	1.75	1.23	0.06
	SD	0.2	0.29	0.11	0.2	0.06	0.07	0.03	0.1	0.16	0.08	0.05
Cl	Mean	1.7	0.52	0.71	1.8	1.74	1.21	0.32	0.5	0.9	0.6	0.26
	Min	0.7	0.18	0.18	0.6	0.93	0.5	0.02	0.1	0.07	0.01	0.13
	Max	2.7	1.42	1.97	2.9	2.86	1.93	1.26	1.4	4.32	2.95	0.4
	SD	0.4	0.46	0.33	0.5	0.49	0.42	0.16	0.3	0.68	0.36	0.13
S	Mean	0.4	0.27	0.29	0.3	0.36	0.31	0.22	0.4	0.26	0.19	0.1
	Min	0.2	0.19	0.17	0.2	0.24	0.23	0.08	0.2	0.05	0.01	0.09
	Max	0.6	0.33	0.45	0.5	0.51	0.37	0.95	0.8	0.72	0.87	0.12
	SD	0.1	0.05	0.06	0.1	0.05	0.04	0.1	0.2	0.11	0.1	0.02
	Mean	33	401	291	305	416	234	24.27	15	144	143	143.8
	Min	−425	223	638	12	130	55.6	−570	−229	−614	−364	118.7
	Max	470	556	7.12	832	873	479	332.5	289	1014	957	182.7
	SD	151	118	174	230	167	127	94.29	131	189	171	40.83
Fe	Mean	177	242	265	312	174	418	129.8	325	332	429	207.2
	Min	64	63	75	87	80	75	38	78	37	32	0
	Max	1230	1000	1620	2000	1990	2720	1160	2290	2950	3000	526.4

SD	151	238	324	381	182	507	93.7	452	342	367	319.2
Zn											
Mean	47	48.2	50.6	31	63.4	30.3	26.54	53	37.5	28.2	29.67
Min	12	29	5	20	25	12	9	26	5	4	0
Max	582	103	142	67	246	74	250	156	294	256	136.4
SD	52	17.1	35.5	9.3	29.7	14.2	16.35	29	26.3	13.5	106.7
Mn											
Mean	36	54.8	60.7	69	69.1	106	105.5	104	93	76.9	31.97
Min	14	34	14	16	16	31	12	22	2	3	14.09
Max	238	114	151	243	277	341	500	497	498	498	49.85
SD	14	19.6	26.9	49	31.7	63.3	79.62	105	71.8	55.3	17.88
Cu											
Mean	8.1	10.5	10.5	7.8	13.4	8.02	7.22	9.5	9.11	8.48	6.21
Min	3	9	3	4	3	2	2	4	2	0	3.57
Max	22	18	24	13	32	22	42	18	49	52	8.85
SD	1.9	2.72	3.79	2.1	5.97	3.6	2.8	2.7	3.55	3.76	2.64
Mo											
Mean	0.9	1.58	2.06	1.8	0.39	1.39	0.73	0.9	1.36	1.29	0.61
Min	0	0.23	0.25	0.1	0	0.05	0	0	0	0	0
Max	4	6.8	6.42	6.3	4.91	4.91	8.68	3.8	10.9	10.8	1.74
SD	0.7	1.53	1.47	1.3	0.63	1.19	0.9	0.9	1.34	1.31	1.13

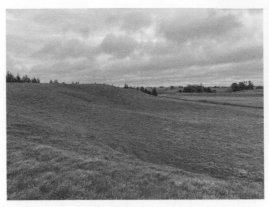

Fig. 8. New Zealand pasture before grazing.

The goal of sampling for the determination of forage being eaten is to mimic the pasture being consumed. In the field, we use the following protocol to obtain a sample of the feed for analysis.

- Evaluate the previous days grazing and compare with the forage to be offered.

It is often possible to evaluate the forage residuals from the previous grazing or day. These are used to evaluate the grazing selection of the cattle (see **Fig. 7**; **Figs. 8–11**). Key points to evaluate how representative a sample is, include.

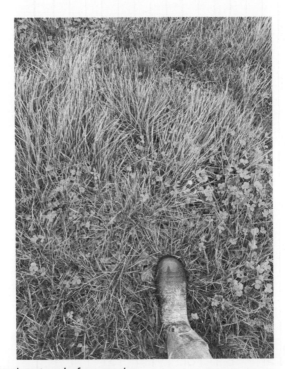

Fig. 9. New Zealand pasture before grazing.

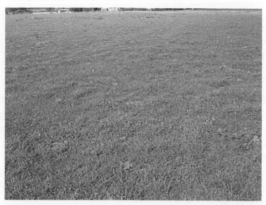

Fig. 10. Mixed pasture that is overgrazed ie the pasture residuals are below the optimum for rapid regrowth.

- History: When was this last grazed, fertilized, or treated with effluent?

These factors will influence a decision about the representative nature of the test. If the sample is being used to determine the suitability of the forage for transition use, the history of fertilizer use either with effluent or fertilizer becomes more critical. The DCAD of forages is greatly impacted by the K content.[15] Soil exposed to manure will increase

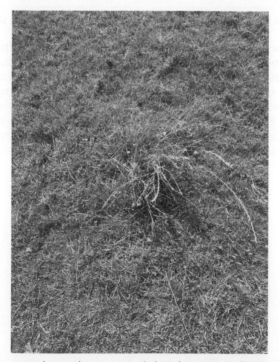

Fig. 11. Cows have grazed very close to an existing dung pat, indicating insufficient availability of pasture. The pasture residuals around the dung pat are too low for optimal regrowth.

in mineral content; quite markedly for some minerals[19]; forages can increase in micronutrient content that are grown on manured soils.[8] Therefore, the pasture sampled needs to be representative of the pastures consumed by the herd or string of cattle for which the diet is being formulated.

- How closely do the cattle graze to the dung pats?

This is an important indicator of grazing pressure and feed availability. Cattle do not graze closely to dung pats unless feed availability is limited (see **Figs. 8** and **9** show pre-grazing pastures and 10 and 11 overgrazed pastures). However, they will select higher, leafy aspects of the sward around dung pats and can graze quite closely to dung pats deposited in a previous rotation (**Figs. 12** and **13**). The closer that cattle graze to the dung pats the higher the N, P, and K content as indicated by similar responses to effluent water.[20] The effects of effluent treatment on increasing DCAD of pastures is well recognized.[21]

Box

Effluent-treated pastures often dramatically increase in DCAD.

- How selective are the cattle and what are they eating?

The comparison of the grazing residuals of recently grazed forages (typically within 5 days) and the forages that they will graze in the coming 5 days allows the selection of a sample that reflects the selective intake.

Box

Examine pastures recently grazed and compare to those about to be grazed (see **Figs. 8–13**).

The examination of residuals can be more important for pastures than for crops that can be sampled by cutting to anticipated or previous grazing height.

The representative sample (approximately 500 g) is taken from at least 10 sites across the grazing area. The larger the area grazed; the more samples required to be representative. We use a plucked sample, or one obtained with pasture (or shearing) shears. For large areas, it is advisable to place the samples into a clean plastic bucket for mixing and sub-sampling. Plastic gloves are recommended for plucking or holding the pasture used for mineral determination.

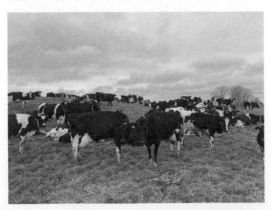

Fig. 12. Cows midway through eating a pasture showing losses due to lying and grazing patterns near dung pats.

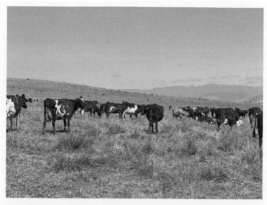

Fig. 13. Cows towards the end of grazing with the residual pasture contrasted between residuals in the dung-pat contaminated areas and areas in between that in which the residuals are low.

The benefit of the plucked sample is being more able to mimic the effect of gripping and tearing pastures, which experience indicates tear near the growth point (**Fig. 14**). The clovers tend to be harvested very close to the ground by cattle. Again, careful observation of the residuals from grazed pasture and comparison with the pasture being sampled is the best guide to the inclusion of clovers or other legumes, herbs, and forbs.

It is difficult to know how much soil should be included in the sample. Cattle ingest considerable amounts of soil when grazing e.g 0.5 to 0.9 kg/d[6,22] and plants with shallow roots will be ingested roots and all! Amounts of soil ingested will be influenced by mud formation and grazing height. Soil ingestion is not exclusive to pasture-fed cattle as cattle in dry lots are often observed to consume soil.

Kao, and colleagues[8] discuss the effects of soil ingestion on sheep nutrition and highlight the interactions among minerals that are likely to influence the uptake of

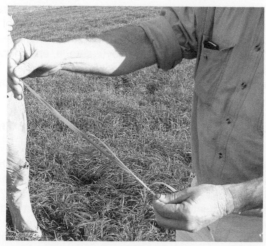

Fig. 14. Showing the growing point of the plant which is circled near the fingers of the left hand.

soil minerals into plants. The range of intakes of Co, Fe, I, Mn, and Se from the soil all exceed that of forage while Cu and Zn intakes from the soil are approximately 50% of the total intake for sheep.[8] It is probable that the contribution of soil mineral to cattle intakes is less because sheep graze pastures lower to the ground than cattle.

Examination of previously grazed areas provides the best indication of soil inges- tion, but caution should be applied as soil mineral content differs markedly from the plant. We typically try to exclude soil, but allow some minor contamination, if this is consistent with the grazing. In dry weather, the plants will often have a dust content; this is consistent with the ingested forage content.

Box

The less the grazing intensity, the more selective cattle will be and the more difficult to obtain a representative sample.

Box

Grazing cattle ingest soil–sometimes quite significant amounts. The mineral content of soil is higher than that of forage.

WHAT FORM ARE THE MINERALS IN?

Considerations of likely risks of deficiency and toxicity will depend on the distribution within the plant e.g.

- Leaf or stem associated,
- Within the cell wall or cytoplasm, and
- Fibre associated or not.

Further, the form of the minerals is also factors that influence the availability of the minerals e.g.

- Ionic,
- Bound in complexes or,
- Amino acid associated including in enzymes.

Minerals in the ionic form are readily available, as are those bound to more ruminally available plant structures such as those in chloroplasts and enzymes, whereas those bound to lignin will be relatively unavailable. Some of the forms of mineral are well recognized as calcium availability is less when bound to oxalates as it is in dock weed (*Rumex spp.*) and some C4 grasses (kikuyu, setaria, and rhodes grass [*Chloris gayana*], paspalum). In contrast, oxalates were not found in ryegrass.[23] See **Table 2** for physical and chemical form of minerals in plants, their sources, and factors influencing availability.

UNDERSTANDING UNCERTAINTY IN MINERAL ASSESSMENT OF CATTLE ON PASTURE

Underwood and Suttle[4] discuss in detail the challenges of evaluating availability of minerals in cattle and note the complexity. The first limitation is determining the amount of minerals ingested and explored in this article. Further, as noted above determining the adequacy of intake is imprecise due to the many different functions of most minerals in cattle and the differing physiological states of the cattle. Cattle have the ability to conserve some minerals and to reduce losses of these. A further complication in evaluating the value of forage and pasture minerals is the availability of the minerals to cattle. It is clear that the form of mineral in the plant will influence

Table 2
Physical and chemical form of minerals in plants and information on the sources and factors influencing the availability

Mineral	Physical and Chemical Form	Sources
Calcium	Essential for plant wall integrity, enzyme function, and signaling. Ca is bound to galacturonic acid in pectin. Is associated with the cell wall especially and vacuole.[24] Forms include calcium phosphate, phytate, ionic calcium, complexed with organic acids,[25] and the much less available oxalate.	Very low concentrations in grains <0.1% and grazing cereals, high in legumes (but availability can be low), C4 grasses can be high in oxalate as can some weeds (dock). Plantain, chicory, soyabean, lablab, and cowpeas are all relatively high in Ca. Calcium in alfalfa and clover is high, but much is fiber associated in the cell wall. Calcium in maize silage is low (see **Table 1**).
Phosphorus	Phosphorus is present as vitamins, mononucleotides, dinucleotides, phsospholipids, phytic acid, sugar phosphates, and lower myo-inositals.[26] A small proportion 3–7% is bound in the cell wall (Whitehead).	Ruminants can use the phytate form of P, much of which is inorganic. Relatively high concentrations are in pastures and grain (often >0.4%). P can be low in some crops eg. bulbs of beets (*Beta vulgaris*).
Sulfur	Sulfur amino acids (cysteine, cystine, and methionine), other organic sulfur-containing compounds (coenzyme A, biotin, and thiamine), sulfate, glutathione, sulfolipids, glycosides, glucosinolates, and thiocyanates.	Note the role for brassicas to have goitrogenic effects and to produce plant toxins (glucosinolates; S-Methyl Cysteine Sulphoxide).[11] Pastures, crops, and grains often exceed 0.1 to 0.2% S
Magnesium	Approximately 50% is water soluble and 10% bound to chlorophyll, some (~10%) is bound to lignin. It is important in enzymatic roles in photosynthesis and protein synthesis.[27]	Most pastures and crops contain >0.15% Mg and grains >0.1%. Availability is influenced by K concentrations, possibly also reduced with increased N availability to pastures. Rapid growth of pastures is associated with low Mg content.
Sodium	Mainly as the ionic form.	Sodium is frequently very low in pastures but can be higher near salt water or around saline soaks. It is important to address Na nutrition for cattle on pastures.
Potassium	Mainly as the ionic form.	Potassium is an important influence on risks of metabolic disease, influencing Ca and Mg metabolism to reduce the availability of these. High concentrations >3.5% are found after fertilization with K fertilizers and after applications of effluent or manure. Urine is high in K. Pastures and crops vary widely in K (see **Table 1**) and grains are often 0.3 to 0.5% K.
Chlorine	Mainly as the ionic form.	Chlorine will increase in pastures and alfalfa with fertilizer application.[28] Pastures and crops vary widely in Cl (see **Table 1**). The uptake of chlorine in the plant can be used to reduce the DCAD. Grains can be <0.1% Cl.

(continued on next page)

Table 2 (continued)

Mineral	Physical and Chemical Form	Sources
Cobalt	Ionic, enzyme associated,[29] in cobalamin.	Regional deficiencies are well-identified and can have a profound effect on animal health and performance. Concentrations are higher in the leaf than the stem in *Trifolium pratense*.[30] Can be increased with fertilization using Co salts and soil is higher in Co than plants. Ingested soil can contribute to Co availability.
Copper	In enzymes that catalyse oxidation involving molecular oxygen. Also, in Cu-protein plastocyanin involved in photosynthesis.[6]	Many pastures are marginal to deficient in Cu (see **Table 1**); however, it is subject to conditioned deficiency from interactions with Fe and especially Mo in the ruminant. Concentrations are higher in the leaf than the stem in *Trifolium pratense*.[30] Legumes are generally higher in Cu than grass.
Iodine	Mainly as the ionic form, iodo-amino acids. Recent evidence supports the potential for I to be essential for plants.	Concentrations increase with plant maturity. Soil ingestion can reduce the risk of I deficiency as the soil is higher in I than the plant. Increased risk of deficiency including clinical goitre on brassica crops e.g. rapes and kales that can contain powerful goitrogens. Alpine valleys are often deficient in I.
Iron	Cytochromes and haem, haemoglobin essential for N fixation by legumes, thiol groups, enzymes[31] particularly oxygen metabolism, porphyrins, and anionic complexes.	Particularly high in soil – contamination will result in high estimates of Fe content. We use high Fe concentrations as an indicator of soil contamination.
Manganese	Electron transfer in redox reactions, enzymes acting as an activator and co-factor for reactions involved in phosphorylation, decarboxylation, and hydrolysis.[32]	Concentrations of Mn in pasture forages often exceed requirements for cattle; however, deficiency can occur. The leaves of alfalfa have more Mn than the stem.[6] Soil contamination can increase test results.
Molybdenum	Anionic form, electron transfer, and enzymatic roles including nitrate reductase. It is essential for N fixation in the rhizobia of legumes.	Concentrations can be high in peat soils >1% and with the use of molybdenized fertilizer used to encourage legume growth.
Selenium	Present as selenate, selenomethionine, and other Se amino acids (selenocysteine) in proteins, dimethylselenide.	Deficiency is common in the Great Plains of North America, New Zealand, Australia, and Scandinavia.
Zinc	Enzymes (dehydrogenases, proteinases, and superoxide dismutase). Stabilizing RNA and DNA structures. Enzymes involved in photosynthesis.[33]	Concentrations of Zn in pasture forages often exceed requirements for cattle (see **Table 1**); however, deficiency can occur. The leaves have higher concentrations than the stem.

The following sources were important in the development of this table.[3–6,18]

Table 3
Mineral supplement options used in pastured herds

Options	Labour	Efficacy
In feed minerals	Minimal for herds that supplementary feed	Provided the mineral formulations are suitable, this is an effective strategy. The distribution of finely powdered products can be a problem, particularly with bridging or with augur systems that can separate fines from more coarse materials. Using pelleted formulations helps avoid sifting and when combined with grains or by-products can ensure palatability.
Minerals in water	Low	Requires monitoring to ensure products are present. Minerals need to be in a soluble form. Potential for interactions with the water source and variable uptake if other water sources are present. Can be very useful in pasture only herds or for heifer groups.
Dusting onto pastures	Minimal	This has been widely used in regions where deficiencies are well known, for example New Zealand. There can be agronomic benefits including increased pasture growth and soil amelioration. It can be difficult for some minerals to supply an adequate amount without substantial wastage.
Boluses	Moderate	While these are often applied infrequently, depending on the length of efficacy, dosing requires some effort. These are a very useful tool for the management of deficiency in pasture only herds or heifer groups. Long duration of action (>100 days) with many formulations.
Free choice minerals (licks or blocks)	Moderate	These can be established in lick feeders or as blocks. Intake is variable, but these are widely used in rangeland situations, often for beef cattle, but are used with dairy heifers and in some milking herds. The block formulations can include urea, ionophores, and other additives; salt is often used as an attractant, but molasses and protein meals are also used. Licks can, similarly, contain additives, be salt, protein or molasses based or simply be a mineral mix. Variability in intake and risks associated with rain are potential limitations to use. Urea toxicity has been noted with rain-affected blocks.
Injectable minerals	Moderate	There is a long history of use with many different formulations. The form of mineral influences the duration of action and distribution of mineral. Some formulations were associated with local irritation and lesions. Some current formulations provide modest increases in mineral status targeted towards periods when requirements for minerals increase. The duration of action varies with the formulation.

availability to the animal and ingestion of mineral-rich soil can influence the availability of minerals. Further, interactions among minerals are well described, such as those among Cu, S, and Mo whereby increased Mo will decrease Cu availability. Similarly, K intake prior to calving results in decreased Ca concentrations after calving. These conditioned deficiencies are well described.

It is important, however, to use a context in which the likelihood of deficiency is identified. Sampling pasture is a vital step in providing evidence that deficiency is likely. This evidence should be combined with health and productivity monitoring, sampling for concentrations in blood, tissue (eg, liver), and milk and observations of response to treatment to identify herds and cattle with mineral deficiency or toxicity states.

Box

Confidence in determining deficiency or toxicity states is achieved by combining feed testing, observations of animal performance and health, animal testing, and responses to treatment.

SUPPLEMENTATION STRATEGIES FOR MINERALS IN PASTURED HERDS

Table 3 provides comments on the strategies available to address mineral deficiencies in pastured herds. Strategies are designed to minimize labor and efficacy of the intervention.

SUMMARY

Given the interactions among minerals, challenges in determining availability, and limitations imposed with soil intake, we can only get an estimate of the availability of minerals to the cow. Sampling pasture mineral content is best done over time to build up a database of concentrations over seasons and with different cultivars.

Pasture mineral testing is an important part of determining the risks of deficiency and toxicity. Building up a picture of the farm by.

- Testing different areas of the farm and different plant species and cultivars provides a context by which to enhance interpretations of clinical observations of cattle production, health, and reproduction.
- Animal testing (blood, tissues, and milk)
- Evaluating responses to intervention provides a better diagnostic basis for evaluating mineral and vitamin status than relying on any of these metrics in isolation.

DISCLOSURES

The authors have nothing to disclose.

SUPPLEMENTARY DATA

Supplementary data related to this article can be found online at https://doi.org/10.1016/j.cvfa.2023.05.003.

REFERENCES

1. National Academies of. Sciences Engineering and Medicine (NASEM). Nutrient requirements of dairy cattle. Eighth revised edition. Washington, DC: The National Academies Press; 2021. https://doi.org/10.17226/25806.2021.
2. Noziere P, Sauvant D, Delaby L. INRA feeding system for ruminants. Wageningen: Wageningen Academic Publishers; 2018.

3. Spears JW. Minerals in forages. In: Fahey G, editor. Forage quality, evaluation, and utilization. American Society of Agronomy; 1994. https://doi.org/10.22134/1994.foragequality.

4. Underwood E, Suttle N. The mineral nutrition of livestock. 3rd edition. Wallingford, UK: CABI; 1999.

5. MacPherson A. Trace-mineral status of forages. In: Givens DI, Owen E, Axford RFE, et al, editors. Forage evaluation in ruminant nutrition. Wallingford, UK: CABI Publishing; 2000. p. 345–71.

6. Whitehead DC. Nutrient elements in grassland: soil-plant-animal relationships. Wallingford, UK: Cabi; 2000.

7. Grace ND. The mineral requirements of grazing ruminants. Palmerston North: Keeling and Mundy Limited, Palmerston North; 1983.

8. Kao PT, Darch T, McGrath SP, et al. Factors influencing elemental micronutrient supply from pasture systems for grazing ruminants. Adv Agron 2020;164: 161–229.

9. Herdt TH, Hoff B. The use of blood analysis to evaluate trace mineral status in ruminant livestock. Vet Clin North Am Food Anim 2011;27(2):255–83.

10. Westwood C, Lean I. Trace elements and vitamin nutrition. Diseases of cattle in australasia—a comprehensive textbook. Wellington: The New Zealand Veterinary Association Foundation for Continuing Education (VetLearnTM); 2010. p. 551–75.

11. Westwood CT. Forages and pastures| annual species and pasture crops – species and varieties. In: McSweeney P, McNamara J, editors. Encyclopedia of dairy sciences. 3rd edition. Elsevier Academic Press; 2021.

12. Moss N. Forages and pastures | annual forage and pasture crops – establishment and management. In: McSweeney P, McNamara J, editors. Encyclopedia of dairy sciences. 3rd edition. Elsevier Academic Press; 2021.

13. Healy W, McCabe W, Wilson G. Ingested soil as a source of microelements for grazing animals. N Z J Agric Res 1970;13(3):503–21.

14. Little D. Studies on cattle with oesophageal fistulae: comparison of concentrations of mineral nutrients in feeds and associated boluses. Aust J Exp Agric 1975;15(75):437–9.

15. Corson D, Waghorn G, Ulyatt M, Lee J. Nirs: Forage analysis and livestock feeding. Paper presented at: Proceedings of the New Zealand Grassland Association1999.

16. Clark D, Mayland H, Lamb R. Mineral analysis of forages with near infrared reflectance spectroscopy. Agron J 1987;79(3):485–90.

17. Clark D, Cary E, Mayland H. Analysis of trace elements in forages by near infrared reflectance spectroscopy. Agron J 1989;81(1):91–5.

18. Little DA. Utilization of minerals. In: Hacker JB, ed. Nutritional limits to animal production from pastures. Proceedings of an international symposium held at St. Lucia, Queensland, Australia, August 24th-28th, 1981: Commonwealth Agricultureal Bureaux, Slough, UK; 1982:259-283.

19. Sheppard S, Sanipelli B. Trace elements in feed, manure, and manured soils. J Environ Qual 2012;41(6):1846–56.

20. Jacobs J, Ward G. Effect of second pond dairy effluent applied in spring to silage regrowth of perennial ryegrass based pasture in southern Australia. 2. Changes in nutritive characteristics and mineral content. Aust J Agric Res 2007;58(2): 145–51.

21. Lean IJ, DeGaris P. Transition cow management: a technical review for nutritional professionals, veterinarians and farm advisors. 2nd edition. Melbourne, Victoria: Dairy Australia; 2021.

22. Healy W. Ingestion of soil by sheep. Paper presented at: N.Z. Soc. Anim. Prod. 1967.
23. Fulkerson W, Slack K, Hennessy D, et al. Nutrients in ryegrass (lolium spp.), white clover (trifolium repens) and kikuyu (pennisetum clandestinum) pastures in relation to season and stage of regrowth in a subtropical environment. Aust J Exp Agric 1998;38(3):227–40.
24. Hirschi KD. The calcium conundrum. Both versatile nutrient and specific signal. Plant Physiol 2004;136(1):2438–42.
25. White PJ, Broadley MR. Biofortification of crops with seven mineral elements often lacking in human diets–iron, zinc, copper, calcium, magnesium, selenium and iodine. New Phytol 2009;182(1):49–84.
26. Frank A. Chemistry of plant phosphorus compounds. Oxford, UK: Elsevier; 2013.
27. Wilkinson S, Welch RM, Mayland H, Grunes D. Magnesium in plants: Uptake, distribution, function, and utilization by man and animals 1990.
28. Goff J, Brummer E, Henning S, et al. Effect of application of ammonium chloride and calcium chloride on alfalfa cation-anion content and yield. J Dairy Sci 2007; 90(11):5159–64.
29. Hu X, Wei X, Ling J, et al. Cobalt: An essential micronutrient for plant growth? Front Plant Sci 2021;1–24.
30. Fleming GA. Mineral composition of herbage. In: Butler GW, Bailey RW, editors. Chemsitry and biochemistry of herbage, vol. 1. London: Academic Press; 1973. p. 529–66.
31. Vigani G, Murgia I. Iron-requiring enzymes in the spotlight of oxygen. Trends Plant Sci 2018;23(10):874–82.
32. Schmidt SB, Husted S. The biochemical properties of manganese in plants. Plants 2019;8(10):381.
33. Brown PH, Cakmak I, Zhang Q. Form and function of zinc plants. Paper presented at: Zinc in Soils and Plants. In: Proceedings of the International Symposium on 'Zinc in Soils and Plants' held at. The University of Western Australia; 1993. p. 27–8.

Trace Mineral Supplementation of Beef Cattle in Pasture Environments

William S. Swecker Jr, DVM, PhD

KEYWORDS

- Cobalt • Copper • Manganese • Zinc • Selenium • Pasture

KEY POINTS

- Free-choice mineral supplements can contain various amounts of macro- and trace minerals, thus careful evaluation of labels is essential to assure the product is meeting the needs of the cattle.
- Intake of mineral supplements is variable, thus measurement of intake is essential to determine the ability of the product to meet the needs of cattle.
- Both Cu and Se deficiencies have been associated with the consumption of endophyte-infected tall fescue.
- Zinc deficiencies have received the most attention relative to trace minerals and bull fertility.

The goal of this article is to present the results of research studies on the challenges when using a free-choice product for trace mineral provision to cows, suckling calves, replacement females, and bulls on patureland as well as special considerations for beef cattle pastured on endophyte-infected tall fescue.[1] The author provides opinions in areas where the literature is lacking. The article concludes with a case study where the intent of supplementation is good but the actual delivery of the trace minerals did not solve the problem.

INTAKE AND FREE-CHOICE MINERALS

When a producer is asked "do the cows have mineral" the author's observation is that a "no" answer is easy to interpret but a "yes" answer can mean plain salt, iodized salt, trace mineral salt, or a salt-mineral mixture. Trace mineral salt is a product that is approximately 95% salt and 5% trace minerals, but there is no specific guidelines on the trace minerals added or the relevant concentrations. A salt-mineral mixture or complete mixture contains the macrominerals such as calcium, phosphorus,

Virginia-Maryland Regional College of Veterinary Medicine, Virginia Tech, 205 Duckpond Drive, Blacksburg, VA 24061-0442, USA
E-mail address: cvmwss@vt.edu

Vet Clin Food Anim 39 (2023) 459–469
https://doi.org/10.1016/j.cvfa.2023.05.004
0749-0720/23/© 2023 Elsevier Inc. All rights reserved.

magnesium, potassium, sodium, and chloride, in addition to trace minerals and vitamins. These products can also be used to deliver compounds beyond macro- and trace minerals. Examples include poloxalene for bloat prevention, insect growth regulators for fly control, antibiotics, and dewormers. Thus, the switching of a product to solve one problem may lead to exacerbation of another problem. Mineral suppliers, however, are required to provide label concentrations, with minimums of all minerals provided and maximums of some. A more detailed description is provided in the introduction article of this series.

EXPECTED INTAKE

There are a limited number of studies where intake of free-choice minerals is compared or reported. Patterson and colleagues[2] reported that mineral intake in fall-calving Angus cows in Kentucky ranged from 95.5 g/day in August to September to 21.5 g/day in December to January with an overall mean of 54.0 g/day over the period of a year. Individual cows varied from 97.3 g/day to 27.9 g/day. The mineral product used in the Patterson study was estimated to contain 24% salt. The investigators noted that the average intake was less than the expected 85 g/day. Pehrson and colleagues[3] reported a mean intake of 110 g/cow/day of a complete mineral (estimated 20% salt) offered to Hereford cows on pasture from mid-March to early June in Sweden. Swecker and colleagues[4] reported a mean intake of 50 g/cow/day of complete mineral (40% salt) from 6 months of gestation (November) to 60 days postpartum (April) in a group of beef cows in Virginia.

Suckling calves will consume mineral mixes before weaning, and recent workers have provided insight on the consumption by cows and their calves. Arthington and colleagues reported intake of fall-calving Brangus cows and their suckling calves in Florida. Calves were an average of 3 months of age, and the project continued until weaning. Average intake for the complete mineral (23% salt) was 65 g/day for the cows and 16 g/d for the calves.[5] Cockwill and colleagues compared mineral intake of Salers cows and calves in Calgary that were first offered a low salt (9.8%NaCl) mineral mix and then a high salt mixture (22.5% NaCl) during July.[6] Consumption by cows was lower for the high salt (183.5 g/d) as compared with the low salt (241.6 g/d) and consumption by calves was 15.7 g/d and 39.3 g/d for high and low salt, respectively. Of note, only 60% of the cows and 23% of the calves visited the feeders during the 1-week observation periods.

These results mirror suggested intakes reported on mineral labels of 56 to 114 g (2–4 oz)/day but also demonstrate that variation is large and some cattle did not consume mineral during observation periods. These results also mirror the anecdotal observation that mineral intake is higher when consuming fresh forage as compared with dormant winter pastures or hay although Manzano and colleagues[7] did not detect a difference in mineral intake of steers between June to July and September to October.

HOW OFTEN DO CATTLE CONSUME FREE-CHOICE MINERAL?

Tait and Fisher reported free-choice mineral intake of Holstein steers offered a mixture of 50% commercial mineral and 50% salt. Average intake was 135 g/steer/day, with a range of 50 to 300 g/steer/day. The steers consumed the mineral on a daily basis, and there was a daily pattern with the largest number of visits to the mineral feeder in the late evening.[8] Manzano and colleagues[7] reported a wide daily variation of individual steers over a 5-day observation period.

Several concepts around free-choice mineral consumption is reflected in these studies. Free-choice mineral consumption does vary within and between herds and animals. Free-choice mineral supplementation works at the level of the pasture group, but one cannot assume that all cattle consumed adequate amounts within a given period. Cattle seem to have an appetite or craving for salt and will consume it at concentrations above their nutrient requirements for sodium or chloride.[9] Domestic ruminants do possess the receptors for the 5 basic tastes with preferences for unami, salt, and sweet, and investigators have proposed that the preference for the salty taste may be positive or negative, depending on the current diet.[10] Anecdotally, small amounts of grain or flavoring agents such as molasses are added to a salt-mineral mixture to enhance intake.

You Need to Monitor Intake!

As a simple example, many salt-mineral products for beef cattle advise an intake of 4 ounces (114 g)/day; this converts to 91 lbs of mineral/cow/year or approximately 2 bags of 50 lb mineral/cow/year or 22 cows/ton of mineral/year. Actual records of mineral feeding can be sparse, but most producers should be able to tell you how many cows are present and how much mineral was purchased. If a producer with 100 cows only purchased 2 tons of mineral, then the problem is availability or provision of the mineral, not the content of the product; this is reinforced by a metabolic profiling study by Macrae and colleagues[11] where they concluded that poor feed intakes or poor feed management were associated with nutritional problems in the herd as compared with poor rations.

TRACE MINERAL SUPPLEMENTATION FOR COW-CALF OPERATIONS
Multiple Minerals

Scientific reports of trace mineral supplementation tend to focus either on biological measures of trace mineral adequacy or on production outcome such as pregnancy rates, calf birth weights, and weaning weights. McDowell and colleagues[12] reported soil, forage, and animal trace mineral concentrations from cows and heifers in 4 regions of Florida. They concluded that trace mineral supplementation was effective in ameliorating deficiencies of Co and partially effective in reducing Cu deficiency based on concentrations of Cu in the liver. The risk of deficiencies in this region was confirmed by Salih and colleagues[13] who reported deficiencies of Cu, Se, and Zn in addition to the micromineral phosphorus in Brahman cattle in sandy soils of central Florida. Harvey and colleagues compared supplementation of sulfate sources of Co, Cu, Zn, and Mn versus organic complexes of the same minerals in Brangus cows from 4 to 9 months of gestation. The cows were fed the supplemental trace minerals as individuals 3 times weekly throughout gestation. Cows fed the sulfate sources did have higher liver concentrations of Cu and Zn at calving, but there was no difference detected in calf production parameters including birth weight or weaning weight. Liver concentrations of Co, Cu, Mn, and Zn were adequate on cows at the initiation of the study.[14] Marques and colleagues[15] compared last trimester supplementation of sulfate sources of Co, Cu, Zn, and Mn versus organic complexes of the same minerals in AngusXHereford cows. The negative control diet was adequate in Co, Cu, Mn, and Zn, and this was reflected by adequate liver concentrations of the same minerals at the initiation of the study. No treatment differences were detected on cow weights or subsequent reproductive performance, and no difference was detected in calf birth weight. Cows that were supplemented did have higher liver Co, Cu, and Zn concentrations in the liver after 75 days as compared with control cows. Calf liver concentrations of Cu and Zn were higher in the cows fed the organic supplement than control cows; calf liver concentrations from the inorganic group were intermediate. A difference in calf birth weight was not detected between treatments; however, calf weaning weight was higher for the calves from cows fed the organic supplement. There were fewer calves from the cows fed organic supplements that were treated for bovine respiratory disease signs during the backgrounding phase than calves from control cows or cows fed inorganic supplements. A treatment effect was not detected for morbidity during the preconditioning phase or finishing phase.

Single Minerals

Rodriguez and colleagues injected parental Cu in late gestation Angus cows in Brazil.[16] The cows were determined to be copper deficient by analysis of serum Cu. They did not detect a difference in birth weight, weaning weight, or subsequent pregnancy rate to fixed time artificial insemination in the cows. The basal forage met the Cu requirements for cows (16.3 ppm Cu), but the forage also contained high concentrations of Mo (5.2 ppm Mo), which likely antagonized Cu absorption. Rowntree and colleagues reported that 20 mg Se given as a weekly drench to Hereford cows in Michigan from first trimester through calving increased plasma Se and erythrocyte glutathione peroxidase in the cows and their calves as compared with control cows with no supplementation. Calf birth weight did not differ between supplemented and control cows.[17] Pehrson and colleagues compared organic and inorganic Se in beef cows. Cow whole blood Se was lower in the inorganic group as compared with the organic group for most periods, but whole blood Se was considered adequate for all groups. Calf whole blood Se was similar at birth among groups, but calves from cows supplemented with organic Se had higher blood Se concentrations than calves from inorganic supplemented dams from months 1 to 6 of age, and whole blood Se of calves from the inorganic supplemented dams was considered marginal at 3 months of age.[2] Selenium is poorly transferred in milk, but organic Se is incorporated into milk in higher concentrations than inorganic Se.[3] Patterson and colleagues compared supplementation with free-choice mineral containing inorganic Se, organic Se, and a mix of both in a year-long study with Angus cows in Kentucky. Pasture Se concentration was less than National Research Council (NRC) recommendations, whereas hay fed during the winter just met the recommendation of 0.1 ppm Se. No difference in calf birth weight, weaning weight, or average daily gain was detected among treatments. Cows and calves from the organic Se treatment group had higher blood Se concentrations for most periods.

BREED DIFFERENCES

Simmental, and possibly Charolais, cattle require higher concentrations of Cu in the ration to maintain adequate Cu status[18,19]; this is possibly due to a lower expression of proteins in the duodenum associated with Cu absorption.[20]

PRE- AND POSTWEANING CALF

Moriel and Arthur offered a limit-fed supplement with and without trace minerals to Brahma–British cross calves for approximately 100 days before weaning in Florida. The study was replicated over 2 years, but the supplement did differ between years. Calves fed supplements with trace minerals had higher concentrations of liver Co, Cu, and Se as compared with calves fed supplement without added trace minerals, but no difference was detected in body weight or gain. They did report that supplement intake was higher in calves offered a supplement without added minerals as compared with the supplement with added minerals in year 1 of the study.[21] A subset of heifer calves were followed-up for 30 days postweaning in the feedlot. No differences in gain or humoral response to porcine red blood cell inoculation was noted between groups. Mattioli and colleagues[22] compared the use of injectable Cu and Zn in Angus heifers in Argentina starting at 3 months of age every 40 days until weaning for a total of 4 injections. The control group was injected with saline. The calves and dams were pastured in a region associated with severe Cu deficiencies and marginal Zn status. The risk of Cu deficiency was confirmed, as the pasture Cu concentrations were less than NRC recommendations, and plasma Cu concentrations were deficient at the initiation of the study. The investigators reported increased body weight, increased hemoglobin, increased packed cell volume, and increased antibody titer to inoculation of BoHV-2 vaccine on days 40 and 80 in the supplemented heifers. Arthington and colleagues[5] reported that the free choice intake of the hydroxychloride forms of Cu, Mn, and Zn was higher than the respective sulfate or organic forms of the same mineral when offered for 18 weeks to preweaned beef calves; however, liver mineral concentration of the calves did not differ between sources in a second phase of the study.

REPLACEMENT FEMALES

Brennan and colleagues[23] reported feeding inorganic Se, organic Se, or a mix of the 2 to Angus-cross replacement heifers in Kentucky. No difference in weight gain or feed between treatments was reported. Although the negative control diet was adequate in Se, supplemented heifers had higher whole blood, plasma, and liver Se as compared with controls. Stokes and colleagues[24] reported the comparison of multiple injections of a combined product that contains Cu, Mn, Se, and Zn with a negative saline control in fall born, commercial Angus heifers from weaning (221 days of age) through pregnancy check after a synchronized artificial insemination (AI). The heifers were pastured on a mix of endophyte-infected tall fescue and red clover pastures and were supplemented with 2.7 kg/day of corn distillers grains. Heifers were provided a free-choice complete mineral, and supplemental injections were given on days 221, 319, 401, and 522. Heifers given the supplemental trace mineral injections had higher plasma Cu, plasma Se, liver Cu, and liver Se than negative control heifers. No difference was detected in body weight, hair coat scores, reproductive tract scores, AI pregnancy rate, or overall pregnancy rate. In a separate study, Stokes and colleagues[25] compared the use of injectable trace minerals at the initiation of a synchronization protocol in heifers with a negative control in a series of 3 experiments. Overall, reproductive outcomes did not differ between the supplemented versus unsupplemented heifers except for a tendency for higher pregnancy rates in the trace mineral–supplemented heifers in Experiment 2. The investigators noted that Angus heifers were used in Experiments 1 and 3, whereas the heifers in Experiment 2 were Simmental X Angus; this may reinforce the concept that Simmentals require more Cu or metabolize Cu and Mn differently than Angus.

REPLACEMENT AND MATURE BULLS

The most critical trace element associated with male infertility is zinc based on rodent work and early work by Pitts who reported decreased testicular size in young Holstein bulls fed a Zn-deficient diet.[26,27] Geary and colleagues compared supplementation of sulfate forms (inorganic) with complexed forms of supplemental Co, Cu, Mn, and Zn in weaned Hereford bull calves.[28] The supplements were fed at approximately 1x, 2x, and 3x times the NRC requirement. Trace mineral supplements were removed from the dams and calves 81 days before the initiation of the study, and the bulls were weaned at 47 days before the initiation of the study. The bulls entered the study at an average of 8.5 months of age, the supplements were fed for 100 days, and a variety of reproductive parameters were measured. Overall, the investigators did not report any differences in reproductive parameters at the P value less than 0.05, but several trends were noted. Bulls supplemented at 3x concentrations with the sulfate form of the minerals had a numerically higher age of puberty than the other groups. All bull groups were Cu-deficient at the initiation of the study based on liver Cu concentrations, and all supplements increased liver Cu to adequate concentrations at day 100 of the study. Liver Zn concentrations decreased in all groups of bulls during the study but remained in the adequate range, and liver Mn concentrations were deficient at the initiation and end of the study. The investigators concluded that the use of complexed forms of Co, Cu, Zn, and Mn may decrease the age of puberty. The numerical difference was 5 days when fed at 1x NRC requirements.

Geary and colleagues[29] followed this study with a 2-year study that compared supplementation with Cu chloride, Zn hydroxychloride, a combination of Cu and Zn, and negative control on weaned Angus bulls in Year 1 and Angus X Hereford bulls in Year 2. The Year 1 bulls were not supplemented with trace minerals for 75 days before the initiation of supplementation and for 120 days on the Year 2. No treatment effect was detected on age at puberty or percentage of bulls that passed a breeding soundness evaluation. Bulls on the control treatment with no Cu or Zn supplementation did have a higher percentage of sperm with a distal midpiece reflection and dag or daglike defects. All bulls were considered Zn adequate in both years of the study. Bulls in Year 1 were Cu-adequate at the initiation of the study and were Cu-deficient in Year 2. Copper supplementation did maintain adequate liver Cu concentrations.

Arthington and colleagues[30] supplemented yearling Angus bulls with inorganic Zn at 40 ppm, a combination of inorganic and organic Zn at 40 ppm and inorganic Zn at 60 ppm for 126 days. Bulls fed the combination of inorganic and organic Zn had a higher percentage of normal sperm than the bulls fed inorganic Zn at 40 ppm. Fewer bulls in the combination group and the 60 ppm Zn group were classified deferred as compared with the 40 ppm Zn inorganic group. Liver Zn concentrations at the end of the study were considered adequate for all groups. Barth and colleagues have proposed that bull nutrition before 26 weeks of age may have a larger impact on subsequent fertility than postweaning diets.[31] This finding may contribute to the lack of consistent results from trace mineral supplementation in postweaning or yearling diets.

Geary and colleagues compared supplementation with sulfate forms of Cu, Mn, and Zn with chloride/hydroxychloride forms of the same minerals and negative control diets in mature beef bulls.[29] A difference in primary reproductive parameters was not detected between supplementation groups. An increase in liver Cu and Zn was observed in the bulls fed the chloride supplement as compared with the sulfate and control groups.

FESCUE

Tall fescue (*Lolium arundinaceum*) infected with the endophyte Epichlöe coenophiala is a common forage plant in many pasture regions in the United States. Production problems have been observed in cattle that consume tall fescue, which include, but are not limited to, decreased growth, decreased pregnancy rates, long hair coats, fat necrosis, and fescue foot.[32] Both Cu and Se deficiencies have been associated with consumption of tall fescue. Dennis and colleagues[33] were the first to report that endophyte-infected fescue had lower Cu concentrations than noninfected fescue both in the greenhouse and pasture. Saker and colleagues reported that serum Cu was lower in steers grazing endophyte-infected fescue than endophyte-free fescue over a 3-year study. Stewart and colleagues[34] reported that liver Cu was lower in steers on endophyte-infected fescue as compared with steers on endophyte free fescue in 1 year of a 2-year study. The investigators attributed the difference to the lower forage intake of the steers on endophyte-infected fescue.

Many soils and forages in the fescue belt are also selenium-deficient. Jia and colleagues[35] reported, through a series of 3 manuscripts, the effects of supplementation with inorganic Se, organic Se, or a 1:1 mixture of inorganic: organic to Angus steers pastured on endophyte-infected fescue pastures in Kentucky. The steers were selected from herds supplemented with the 3 methods of Se supplementation noted earlier, were fed no supplemental Se for a 97-day depletion period where they were acclimated to pasture Calan gates, and then went through an 86-day grazing trial where they were individually offered 1 of the 3 Se supplements. Whole-blood Se concentrations were higher in the organic and mixture groups as compared with the inorganic group; however, blood Se concentrations were adequate in all groups. Serum prolactin decreased in all steers while on the endophyte-infected fescue but were higher for the organic and mixed groups than the inorganic groups. Hepatic glutamine synthetase messenger RNA activity and protein content were higher for the organic and mixed groups than the inorganic groups.[35] Serum albumin was higher in steers fed the mixed form of Se, and serum alkaline phosphatase was higher in steers fed the mixed form and organic forms of Se. Both of these measures tend to be decreased in cattle affected by fescue toxicosis.[36] Steers were harvested at the end of the study, and Li and colleagues[37] measured gene expression in the pituitary. Steers in the mixed Se group and organic Se group had higher prolactin synthetic potential through separate pathways. Webb and colleagues compared the use of the inorganic/organic mix with inorganic Se on steers grazed on endophyte-infected and endophyte-free fescue pastures in a 2X2 design. Steers offered the inorganic/organic mix of Se had increased serum prolactin compared with steers offered inorganic Se, but prolactin concentrations were not as high as steers on endophyte-free fescue. The investigators concluded that the use of the mix of inorganic/organic Se as a supplement partially ameliorated the negative effects of endophyte-infected fescue.

In summary, increased attention to Cu and Se supplementation is warranted for cattle that consume endophyte-infected tall fescue.

CASE STUDY

A commercial Angus herd of approximately 200 head was challenged with Se deficiency/white muscle disease in neonatal calves, which was supported by laboratory diagnosis. The nutrition advisor instituted a trace mineral salt mixture with Se as a sole source of minerals to the cows in response to the cases. During the next calving season, clinical cases of hypomagnesemia were observed, thus the next response was to add a macro/trace mineral–combined product with 10% magnesium. A divider was placed in the mineral feeders, with the high magnesium mineral on one side and the trace mineral salt with Se on the other (**Fig. 1**).

As the herd moved to the next calving season, cases of Se deficiency and hypomagnesemia were recorded. The critical error, in the author's opinion, was to give the cows the option to choose one mineral or the other rather than developing or purchasing a high magnesium mineral with added Se or at least mix the 2 products. This concept reinforces the challenge of assuring that the client understands the critical nutrients provided by the supplements, and fixing one problem may lead to another. Another example is dealing with bloat due to excessive clover in a given year. An immediate response would be to switch to bloat blocks, which can help with the immediate

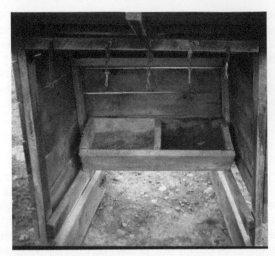

Fig. 1. Mineral feeder from case study. The product on the left is a high-Magnesium salt-mineral mixture but does not contain adequate Se. The product on the right is a trace mineral salt with Se. Reliance on the cows to consume both products failed.

problem of bloat but may result in longer term deficiencies of trace minerals that are not provided in the same amount in the bloat blocks as the previous mineral.

SUMMARY

Cow-calf production systems in pasture environments are at risk for one or more trace mineral deficiencies, especially when a supplementation program is absent or inadequate. The provision of trace minerals through either a trace mineralized salt or a complete mineral works at the herd level, but the practitioner and client must recognize the variation in intake among cows and calves. This variation is reflected when sampling plasma or liver concentrations within a group or herd, and thus the use of mean concentrations of the group should be used to reflect the herd's status. The reader may have noticed that most of the studies focus on Cu, Mn, Zn, and Se provided either in combination or singularly. Supplementation of Cu, Zn, and Se repeatedly increase the mineral status of the animal as measured by blood/plasma or liver; however, the production benefit of the increase is inconsistent. Manganese is still confusing to the author, as the response to supplementation seems many times to be inconsistent or negligible. The trace minerals Co, I, and Fe are rarely evaluated, which suggests that common feeds or supplements provide adequate supply.

As a nutritionist, the author suggests that the first step in planning mineral supplementation program or determination of the role of trace minerals in a production or disease challenge is to consider the trace mineral content of the basal feeds, which can reveal both deficiencies or the presence of high concentrations of antagonists; this is followed by assessment of both the trace mineral content and intake of supplements. At this point, sampling of the animals in question may be warranted to assure either the adequate provision of the trace element or their role in the current production problem. Pulse dosing via injections or oral products may be used to provide additional nutrients in time of need.

The reader may find a review of the literature confusing, as outcomes can be inconsistent. The author suggests you consider the following when evaluating either research studies or outcomes in their clients' herds.

1. What is the status of the animals at the initiation and the end of the trial? Deficient, marginal, adequate?
2. What is the goal of supplementation? To correct the deficient state, to maintain the adequate state, to increase pregnancy rates, to decrease disease incidence?

The reader probably recognizes that supplementation studies generally will result in increased concentrations of the mineral in liver or blood/plasma, especially in deficient animals. A consistent and repeatable change in pregnancy rates or growth rates is not found across all studies and in the same way is unlikely to be found across all herds served by a clinician. Provision of trace mineral supplements, however, is a risk management tool to promote productivity. The program can be fine-tuned, on a cost-effective basis, with the knowledge of the trace mineral concentrations of the common feeds in the region and determination of the needed outcomes.

DISCLOSURE

No current conflicts to disclose.

FUNDING

2022 NAHMS Bison study cooperative agreement: Funded by USDA APHIS and Forage Work Plan.

REFERENCES

1. National Resources Inventory (NRI) Glossary. Secondary National Resources Inventory (NRI) Glossary 2015. Available at: https://www.nrcs.usda.gov/sites/default/files/2022-10/NRI_glossary.pdf. Accessed June 21, 2023.
2. Patterson JD, Burris WR, Boling JA, et al. Individual intake of free-choice mineral mix by grazing beef cows may be less than typical formulation assumptions and form of selenium in mineral mix affects blood se concentrations of cows and their suckling calves. Biol Trace Elem Res 2013;155(1):38–48.
3. Pehrson B, Ortman K, Madjid N, et al. The influence of dietary selenium as selenium yeast or sodium selenite on the concentration of selenium in the milk of Suckler cows and on the selenium status of their calves. J Anim Sci 1999; 77(12):3371–6.
4. Swecker WS Jr, eversole DE, Thatcher CD, et al. Selenium supplementation of gestating beef cows on selenium-deficient pastures. Agri Pract 1991;12(2): 25–30.
5. Arthington JD, Silveira ML, Caramalac LS, et al. Effects of varying sources of Cu, Zn, and Mn on mineral status and preferential intake of salt-based supplements by beef cows and calves and rainfall-induced metal loss. Transl Anim Sci 2021; 5(2):txab046 [published Online First: 20210307].
6. Cockwill C, McAllister T, Olson M, et al. Individual intake of mineral and molasses supplements by cows, heifers and calves. Canadian Journal of Animal Science - CAN J ANIM SCI 2000;80:681–90.
7. Manzano RP, Paterson J, Harbac MM, et al. The effect of season on supplemental mineral intake and behavior by grazing steers. Prof Anim Sci 2012;28(1):73–81.
8. Tait RM, Fisher LJ. Variability in individual animal's intake of minerals offered free-choice to grazing ruminants. Anim Feed Sci Technol 1996;62(1):69–76.
9. Berger L.L., Salt and Trace Minerals for Livestock, Poultry, and Other Animals. 2006.

10. Ginane C, Baumont R, Favreau-Peigné A. Perception and hedonic value of basic tastes in domestic ruminants. Physiol Behav 2011;104(5):666–74 [published Online First: 2011/07/30].

11. Macrae AI, Whitaker DA, Burrough E, et al. Use of metabolic profiles for the assessment of dietary adequacy in UK dairy herds. Vet Rec 2006;159(20):655–+.

12. McDowell LR, Kiatoko M, Bertrand JE, et al. Evaluating the nutritional status of beef cattle herds from four soil order regions of Florida. II. Trace minerals. J Anim Sci 1982;55(1):38–47 [published Online First: 1982/07/01].

13. Salih YM, McDowell LR, Hentges JF, et al. Mineral status of grazing beef cattle in the warm climate region of Florida. Trop Anim Health Prod 1983;15(4):245–51 [published Online First: 1983/11/01].

14. Harvey KM, Cooke RF, Colombo EA, et al. Supplementing organic-complexed or inorganic Co, Cu, Mn, and Zn to beef cows during gestation: physiological and productive response of cows and their offspring until weaning. J Anim Sci 2021;99(5). https://doi.org/10.1093/jas/skab095.

15. Marques RS, Cooke RF, Rodrigues MC, et al. Effects of organic or inorganic cobalt, copper, manganese, and zinc supplementation to late-gestating beef cows on productive and physiological responses of the offspring. J Anim Sci 2016; 94(3):1215–26 [published Online First: 2016/04/12].

16. Rodríguez AM, López Valiente S, Mattioli G, et al. Effects of inorganic copper injection in beef cows at late gestation on fetal and postnatal growth, hematology and immune function of their progeny. Res Vet Sci 2021;139:11–7.

17. Rowntree JE, Hill GM, Hawkins DR, et al. Effect of Se on selenoprotein activity and thyroid hormone metabolism in beef and dairy cows and calves. J Anim Sci 2004;82(10):2995–3005.

18. Ward JD, Spears JW, Gengelbach GP. Differences in copper status and copper metabolism among angus, simmental, and charolais cattle. J Anim Sci 1995; 73(2):571–7 [published Online First: 1995/02/01].

19. Pogge DJ, Richter EL, Drewnoski ME, et al. Mineral concentrations of plasma and liver after injection with a trace mineral complex differ among Angus and Simmental cattle. J Anim Sci 2012;90(8):2692–8.

20. Fry RS, Spears JW, Lloyd KE, et al. Effect of dietary copper and breed on gene products involved in copper acquisition, distribution, and use in angus and simmental cows and fetuses. J Anim Sci 2013;91(2):861–71 [published Online First: 20121112].

21. Moriel P, Arthington JD. Effects of trace mineral-fortified, limit-fed preweaning supplements on performance of pre- and postweaned beef calves. J Anim Sci 2013;91(3):1371–80.

22. Mattioli GA, Rosa DE, Turic E, et al. Effect of Injectable Copper and Zinc Supplementation on Weight, Hematological Parameters, and Immune Response in Preweaning Beef Calves. Biol Trace Elem Res 2019;189(2):456–62 [published Online First: 20180908].

23. Brennan K, Burris W, Boling J, et al. Selenium content in blood fractions and liver of beef heifers is greater with a mix of inorganic/organic or organic versus inorganic supplemental selenium but the time required for maximal assimilation is tissue-specific. Biol Trace Elem Res 2011;144(1–3):504–16.

24. Stokes RS, Volk MJ, Ireland FA, et al. Effect of repeated trace mineral injections on beef heifer development and reproductive performance. J Anim Sci 2018; 96(9):3943–54 [published Online First: 2020/05/22].

25. Stokes RS, Ralph AR, Mickna AJ, et al. Effect of an injectable trace mineral at the initiation of a 14 day CIDR protocol on heifer performance and reproduction1. Translational Animal Science 2017;1(4):458–66.
26. Pitts WJ, Miller WJ, Fosgate OT, et al. Effect of zinc deficiency and restricted feeding from two to five months of age on reproduction in holstein bulls1. J Dairy Sci 1966;49(8):995–1000.
27. Hidiroglou M. Trace element deficiencies and fertility in ruminants: a review. J Dairy Sci 1979;62(8):1195–206 [published Online First: 1979/08/01].
28. Geary TW, Kelly WL, Spickard DS, et al. Effect of supplemental trace mineral level and form on peripubertal bulls. Anim Reprod Sci 2016;168:1–9 [published Online First: 20160220].
29. Geary TW, Waterman RC, Van Emon ML, et al. Effect of supplemental trace minerals on standard and novel measures of bull fertility. Theriogenology 2021;172: 307–14 [published Online First: 20210716].
30. Arthington JD, Corah LR, Hill DA. The effects of dietary zinc concentration and source on yearling bull growth and fertility11contribution no. R-08583 from the florida agriculture experiment station. Prof Anim Sci 2002;18(3):282–5.
31. Barth AD, Brito LF, Kastelic JP. The effect of nutrition on sexual development of bulls. Theriogenology 2008;70(3):485–94 [published Online First: 2008/06/10].
32. Roberts C, Andrae J. Tall fescue toxicosis and management. Crop Manag 2004; 3(1). https://doi.org/10.1094/cm-2004-0427-01-mg.
33. Dennis SB, Allen VG, Saker KE, et al. Influence of Neotyphodium coenophialum on copper concentration in tall fescue. J Anim Sci 1998;76(10):2687–93.
34. Stewart RL, Scaglia G, Abaye OA, et al. Tall fescue copper and copper-zinc superoxide dismutase status in beef steers grazing three different fescue types. Prof Anim Sci 2010;26(5):489–97.
35. Jia Y, Li Q, Burris WR, et al. Forms of selenium in vitamin-mineral mixes differentially affect serum prolactin concentration and hepatic glutamine synthetase activity of steers grazing endophyte-infected tall fescue. J Anim Sci 2018;96(2): 715–27.
36. Jia Y, Son K, Burris WR, et al. Forms of selenium in vitamin-mineral mixes differentially affect serum alkaline phosphatase activity, and serum albumin and blood urea nitrogen concentrations, of steers grazing endophyte-infected tall fescue. J Anim Sci 2019;97(6):2569–82.
37. Li Q, Jia Y, Burris WR, et al. Forms of selenium in vitamin-mineral mixes differentially affect the expression of genes responsible for prolactin, ACTH, and alpha-MSH synthesis and mitochondrial dysfunction in pituitaries of steers grazing endophyte-infected tall fescue. J Anim Sci 2019;97(2):631–43.

Trace Mineral Supplementation for Beef Cows: Dry Range Environment

Bob Sager, DVM, PhD[a],*, Robert J. Van Saun, DVM, MS, PhD[b]

KEYWORDS

- Trace minerals • Requirements • Mineral interactions • Beef cattle
- Dry range conditions

KEY POINTS

- Trace minerals play important biologic roles in supporting cow and calf health, productivity, and support of immune function.
- Range forages do not adequately supply sufficient essential trace minerals to meet requirements for beef cattle in differing physiologic states.
- Free choice mineral supplementation is the most economic, practical method for grazing herds; however, a disadvantage is the lack of uniform consumption by animals.
- For commercial mineral supplements, "one product does not fit each operation," and modern beef production requires supplemental mineral nutrition for meet requirements for animal health and performance.
- Forage testing may not always be practical under range conditions; thus, assessment of animal trace mineral status is necessary to monitor supplementation outcome.

INTRODUCTION

Beef cattle grazing native forage in range environments is unique in livestock production. The ability to use these forages is due to the synergistic relationship between host ruminant and rumen microbes, which allows range forage to be converted into high-quality microbial protein and non-tillable land to be used for animal production. Utilization of range forage is considerably variable with demands dependent on class of cattle using the range, desired production, and economical influence affecting use and production goals. Trace minerals are necessary for both microbial growth and reproduction and required by the host bovine for various metabolic, antioxidant,

[a] Medicine Creek Bovine Health and Consulting, PO Box 614, White Sulphur Springs, MT 59645, USA; [b] Department of Veterinary and Biomedical Sciences, College of Agricultural Sciences, Pennsylvania State University, 108C Animal, Veterinary and Biomedical Sciences Building, University Park, PA 16802-3500, USA
* Corresponding author.
E-mail address: hammerbeef.sager97@gmail.com

Vet Clin Food Anim 39 (2023) 471–489
https://doi.org/10.1016/j.cvfa.2023.08.012
0749-0720/23/© 2023 Elsevier Inc. All rights reserved.

and immunologic functions.[1-3] Trace mineral nutrition in beef cattle production is obtained through grazing primary forages and additional supplemental trace minerals to achieve desired requirements to support production goals, health, and performance. This interaction between trace mineral requirements and beef cattle production is complex and not fully elucidated. Many factors influence trace mineral supplementation response such as dietary mineral concentration, cow physiologic state, presence or absence of trace mineral antagonists, soil, water, or environmental factors, and other complex animal factors including performance goals, stress conditions, and host tissue absorption and metabolism.[3-5] The objective of this article is to provide a basic understanding of trace mineral needs as influenced by mineral interactions and supplementation practices for beef cattle managed in dry range conditions typical of the western United States.

TRACE MINERAL REQUIREMENTS AND DISEASE

Minerals are classified into two broad groups: macrominerals and microminerals. Macrominerals, namely calcium (Ca), phosphorus (P), magnesium (Mg), potassium (K), sodium (Na), chloride (Cl), and sulfur (S), are those required in amounts greater than 1000 mg per day for normal growth, production, and reproduction. Microminerals, namely chromium (Cr), cobalt (Co), copper (Cu), iodine (I), iron (Fe), manganese (Mn), molybdenum (Mo), selenium (Se), and zinc (Zn), are those required in milligram (mg) or nanogram (ng) amounts per day. Beef cattle trace mineral requirements were first published by the National Research Council (NRC; now termed National Academies of Science, Engineering and Medicine [NASEM]) in the 1950s when production requirements for beef cattle production were two-thirds of present day production expectations.[6] Recommended NRC trace mineral requirements were derived from experiments during the 1950s using cattle that were genetically different, raised with a different production focus, and fed different diets. Subsequent NRC publications in 1984, 1996, 2000 (update), and 2016 continued to modify beef cattle requirements based on current published data; however, there are minimal changes in trace mineral requirements over this period (**Table 1**).[3,7-9] The NASEM (2016) addresses 17 minerals required for beef cattle production; however, no definitive requirements were determined for Mo, nickel, and Cr.[3] Biologic functions of the trace minerals is described elsewhere in this issue[10] and in various texts.[5,11]

Trace Mineral Diseases

As with any essential nutrient, mineral-associated nutritional disease is a consequence of either deficient availability or excessive amounts relative to requirement leading to mineral-specific deficiency or toxicosis clinical signs.[5] Trace mineral toxicosis diseases are discussed elsewhere in this issue.[12] Range beef cattle have the greatest risk for Se intoxication within certain geographic regions from consuming indicator (ie, *Astragalus bisulcatus*) or secondary (ie, native range forages, wheatgrass, barley, alfalfa) Se-accumulating forages.[13,14] Chronic Se-toxicosis inducing the disease entity of "blind staggers" has been questioned and related more to sulfur toxicosis.[15] Other trace mineral toxicities most likely are a result of improper supplementation practices.

Mineral deficiencies are increasingly more important now than in the past because of the magnified importance of the economic production focus of animal production. Clinical mineral deficiencies and imbalances for cattle are reported from all regions of the world.[5,11] A variety of mineral elements are likely to be lacking under normal

Table 1
Comparison of recommended dietary trace mineral requirements (mg/kg dietary dry matter) for beef cattle from the 1958 to 2016 National Research Council publications for beef cattle nutrient requirements[3,6–9]

Trace Mineral	1958[b]	1984[c]	2000 Update[d]	2016[d]	Stressed Calves[e]
Cobalt	0.07–0.11	0.1 (0.07–0.11)	0.07–0.11	0.15	0.1–0.2
Copper	4–8	8 (4–10)	10 (4–15)	10 (4–15)	10–15
Chromium	ND	ND	ND (0.2–1)	ND (0.2–1)	ND
Iron	<33	50 (50–100)	50	40–50	100–200
Iodine	0.4–0.8	0.5 (0.2–2.0)	0.5	0.5	0.3–0.6
Manganese	6.6–11	40 (20–50)	20–40	20–40	40–70
Molybdenum	ND	ND	ND	ND	ND
Selenium[a]	ND	0.2 (0.05–0.3)	0.1	0.1	0.1–0.2
Zinc	ND	30 (20–40)	30	30	75–100

[a] Selenium supplementation is restricted by the Food and Drug Administration to 3 mg/day or 0.3 mg/kg dietary dry matter for beef cattle.
[b] ND = no requirement was determined. Considered dietary forage sufficient to provide. Iron requirement based on swine. Selenium was only considered toxic and not required.
[c] Table 4 in NRC, 1984, provides a suggested value and (range) for each mineral. The range is recognizing various dietary and animal factors that could impact the actual dietary requirement.
[d] A range for dietary copper concentration was provided to account for presence of sulfur (<0.25%) and molybdenum (<2 mg/kg) in the diet. Data suggesting chromium does provide some benefit were suggested but insufficient data were available to define a requirement.
[e] Increased dietary mineral concentrations suggested for stressed calves from the NASEM, 2016 report.[3]

grazing conditions for ruminants (**Box 1**).[3,16] With attention to productive efficiency, the prevalence of clinical deficiency diseases has been greatly reduced. A greater issue is what is termed subclinical deficiency (or toxicosis) with nonspecific impacts on productive efficiency.[17–19] Marginal trace mineral deficiencies are associated with reduced growth rates, impaired reproduction, and greater disease susceptibility resultant from impaired immune function.[16,20] This situation is most pertinent to calves and the potential stress they will be exposed too following weaning and transportation to feeding enterprises.[21,22] The need for additional trace minerals for stressed calves is recognized in suggested requirements in the NASEM (2016) report (see **Table 1**).[3]

Box 1
Mineral elements most likely to be deficient under grazing conditions

- Calcium
- Phosphorus
- Sodium
- Cobalt
- Copper
- Iodine
- Selenium
- Zinc

RANGE CATTLE TRACE MINERAL CONSIDERATIONS

Daily nutritional status of beef cattle has important implications for productive outputs including maintenance, growth, lactation, and reproduction. Maintenance is considered the largest component of the trace mineral requirement and often related to dry matter intake.[3] Unlike the current NASEM dairy cattle publication, beef cattle mineral requirements, other than Ca and P, are not factorially derived but based on a recommended dietary concentration (mg/kg = parts per million [ppm]). First and most important is the fact that mineral requirements vary greatly with many factors (**Box 2**). Using a dietary concentration to define trace mineral needs relies on the animal consuming sufficient dietary dry matter to consume an appropriate mineral mass to meet biologic needs. Seasonal differences, differences of farm or ranch availability, ecosystem influences, and different management systems have large influences in availability and intake that change requirements of supplemented minerals for desired production.

Breed and Genetic Implications

Consideration of how trace mineral nutrition has changed is reflective on how beef cattle genetics have changed in the past 100 years (**Fig. 1**). One might surmise modern beef cow genetics require increased trace mineral nutrition to meet genetic potential and achieve desired performance. In the past 50 years, US beef cattle productive efficiency has increased nearly 50% due to improved genetics, advances in nutrition, biotechnology, advances in animal health, and value-added management.[23] More productive continental breeds have higher requirements compared with traditional British breeds. Simmental cattle had greater biliary Cu excretion compared with Angus cattle.[24] Angus cattle had improved Cu status compared with Charolais and Simmental cattle consuming the same diet.[25] Further investigation into transporter mechanisms showed Simmental cattle to be less efficient with intestinal Cu absorption compared with Angus cattle.[26] Only recently has recommended Co requirement been increased due to genetic production needs.[27] Today beef cattle production involves animals that are 35% to 40% larger anatomically, grow at increased rates, and are developed with more focus on muscle growth with efficient gain than 50 years ago thus the potential for increased trace mineral requirements. Most nutrient recommendations are not based on an immunologic or health status endpoint; increased requirements for trace minerals may be required for genetic potential and critical for the health in beef cattle production.

Trace Mineral Interactions

Dietary minerals can be altered in the rumen environment or interact with each other at the level of the intestine to reduce availability.[28,29] Many interactions have not been

---

Box 2
Factors affecting trace mineral requirements

- Animal physiologic state, production level
- Geographic location
- Geologic soil mineral differences
- Water source total dissolved solids (TDS)
- Weather and environmental factors
- Related stresses that require additional intake to meet requirements

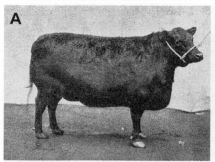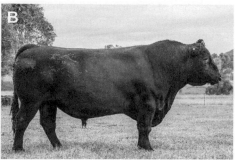

Fig. 1. Comparison of the change in Angus cattle conformation obtained through genetic selection. (A) An antique photo of an Angus cow in the early 1900's. (B) A current day Angus bull. ([A] Photo credit: iStock with permission; [B] https://www.istockphoto.com/photo/angus-cattle-gm1401813903-454931047 with permission.)

characterized, and multiple interactions between different minerals make availability difficult to estimate requirements.[30] The association of minerals with fiber fractions in feedstuffs and/or binding of minerals to undigested fiber constituents in the gastrointestinal tract may alter bioavailability of some trace minerals in ruminants.[11]

The well-characterized mineral interaction in ruminants is that between Cu, Mo, and S.[31–34] Forage Cu content west of the Mississippi River is generally lower than the eastern part of the United States.[35–38] Sulfates in water or feed can be especially problematic with trace mineral availability as sulfate is converted to the sulfide anion, which can combine with most cations forming an insoluble sulfide compound. The relationship between Mo and S in the rumen as well as rumen pH will direct the formation of various thiomolybdate compounds.[31] Higher molar ratio of S:Mo with lower rumen pH induces predominately tetrathiomolybdate formation, which is the most potent Cu chelator. Thiomolybdate compounds can be absorbed and then capable of binding to Cu in proteins reducing their functionality.[31]

The initial description of mineral interactions was direct interactions, either antagonistic or synergistic, between various minerals in support of plant or animal metabolism. This interaction of "mineral wheel" may include only essential or essential and toxic minerals. This perspective does not address recognized three-way mineral interactions. Iron can further contribute to the thiomolybdate–Cu interaction, but not directly with Cu.[31] Iron status is influenced by Cu deficiency but only with elevated Mn status.[30] Other more complex mineral interactions remain to be identified.

Is Availability Important?

Most minerals are absorbed in the duodenum through the interaction of water-soluble metal ion with specific or nonspecific metal transporters located in the brush border.[28,39] Mineral transporters are specific to the metal ion valence, for example, Cu is only absorbed by its transporter protein (Cu-transporter 1) when in the +1 state.[28,39] Minerals are not absorbed across the gut mucosa bound to a ligand. The evaluation of Zn absorption from differing sources (inorganic and Zn-methionine) showed no significant differences in availability and no indication of labeled methionine absorption.[40] The only exception here is the organic form of Se, namely selenomethionine. In this molecule, the S atom is replaced by Se given the two molecules have very similar chemical properties. Selenium availability is generally reported to be greater with selenomethionine compared with inorganic forms.[41,42] The greater incorporation of Se into body and milk proteins is suggestive of selenomethionine being absorbed by the amino acid transporter.

As impact of the rumen environment on inorganic mineral sources has been identified, the use of organic or chelated mineral sources has been used to improve mineral availability.[43,44] Metal cations can be linked to amino acid, peptide, hydrolyzed protein, polysaccharide, or other carbohydrate ligands.[45] Hydroxylated minerals are a more recent addition to mineral supplements and seem to have a similar rumen protective effect on the metal cation.[39] The metal cation can be bound by coordinate covalent bond, ionic associations, or covalent bonds forming heterocyclic rings (chelates).[46] The stability constant is a measure of the affinity between a metal ion and its ligand. Under the acidic conditions of the abomasum, the metal-ligand complex dissociates or solubilizes.[28] If the ligand does not solubilize, dissociate, or is too large to pass through cellular tight junctions, mineral ion bioavailability will be reduced. Organic mineral sources come with a higher expense and supplementing higher levels of inorganic mineral sources often results in similar cow response. Peer-reviewed information should be critically evaluated in deciding on use of organic minerals and expected returns on investment.

DIETARY TRACE MINERAL INTAKE

Consumed mineral can come from three primary sources in the grazing beef cattle diet: pasture or harvested forages, supplements (ie, commercial or farm-mixed protein, energy supplements with minerals and vitamins; free choice minerals), and water. The determination of total mineral intake will depend on the accuracy of mineral content assessment of each of the dietary components.

Forage Mineral

Cattle derive a large proportion of their consumed mineral from forages during grazing. Mineral content is highly dependent on vegetative components and seeds of specific forages and associated grains consumed. Plant mineral content is regulated by both external and internal factors. Concentrations are dependent on plant genus and species, soil type on which the plant grows, climatic conditions (ie, daylength, ambient temperature, precipitation) during growth, and plant stage of maturity when consumed.[47] Soil pH is an important factor in plant mineral content. Macrominerals generally are taken up by plants more efficiently in neutral soil conditions; hence, the use of liming to acidic soils.[47] In contrast, most trace minerals are absorbed by plants more efficiently under acidic soil conditions. An exception here is Mo, which is absorbed more efficiently under neutral soil conditions.[48]

Although forage is a primary contributor to dietary mineral, its contribution is highly variable under range grazing conditions given the potential wide variety of vegetative material consumed in a geographic region. One large study focused on forage mineral content for feeding beef cattle determined mineral content from 709 forage samples from 23 states finding a high prevalence of deficiencies in Cu, Se, and Zn.[37] In this survey, the investigators interpreted determined forage trace mineral content into categories of deficient, marginally deficient, and adequate relative to NRC (1996) defined beef cattle requirements (**Table 2**). Criteria used would be considered conservative in comparison to current beef cattle trace mineral requirements suggesting a greater prevalence of marginal and deficient forages (**Table 3**).

Forage nutrient content assessment is a foundational component of the nutrition program. The National Forage Testing Association (www.foragetesting.org) provides information on obtaining representative samples for testing, forage probes for sampling, and a listing of certified laboratories. Sampling and testing harvested forage

Table 2
Criteria used by Mortimer et al (1999) for characterizing forage mineral content relative to National Research Council (1996) beef cattle mineral requirements[8,37]

Trace Mineral	Deficient Status	Marginally Deficient	Adequate
Copper	<4 ppm	4–9.9 ppm	≥10 ppm
Manganese	<20 ppm	20–39.9 ppm	≥40 ppm
Selenium	<0.1 ppm	0.1–0.199 ppm	≥0.2 ppm
Zinc	<20 ppm	20–29.9 ppm	≥30 ppm
Copper:molybdenum ratio	<4:1	4.0–4.5:1	>4.5–5:1

			Antagonistic Level	
Copper Antagonists	Deficient	Ideal	Marginal	High
Iron	<50 ppm	50–200 ppm	>200–400 ppm	>400 ppm
Molybdenum	NA	<1.0 ppm	1–3 ppm	> 3 ppm
Sulfur	< 0.10%	0.15%–0.20%	>0.2%–0.3%	> 0.3%

or improved pasture is reasonably straightforward. Collecting forage samples in an extensive grazing system is problematic and may not be feasible to accurately assess what the cows are consuming. Many western US extension services and the NASEM (2016) have native range forage composition data, but these data may be limited in numbers and trace mineral information.[3,35] Tabular data should be used sparingly as it may not be representative of a given geographic region. Some forage laboratories compile their data that can be sorted by forage type, location, year, and nutrients of interest. If an appropriate sample can be collected be sure the minerals are determined by wet chemistry methods and not near-infrared spectroscopy.[49] The typical trace minerals measured are Fe, Cu, Mn, and Zn. Most laboratories will offer S, Mo, and Se as additional cost items for analysis. Selenium analysis is quite expensive and should only be used in regions of toxicity or deficiency concerns, or to establish Se status for your region.

Water

Water is considered a most essential nutrient and evaluated relative to its availability and quality. An often-overlooked area is water evaluation as water is the largest single nutrient and water quality can vary greatly even on the same production unit.[50] Water analysis can vary on the same ranch often only short distances apart. Soil and water mineral contents will vary during drought and reservoir total dissolved solids (TDS) will vary after rainfalls of 0.5 inches or more after runoff has accumulated. Water can contain a significant amount of dissolved substances measured as (TDS) or salinity.[51] Various university extension services provide livestock water quality assessment information.[52,53] Minerals dissolved in water are readily available and will contribute to total mineral intake. Water-associated minerals may include those contributing to required minerals, antagonistic agents to minerals, and toxic minerals.[51] Elevated water saline will reduce feed intake and often this is associated with high soluble sulfates that will interfere with Se and Cu availability.[54] Excessive sulfur intake could lead to toxicosis and "blind staggers" and polioencephalomalacia.[15,54] Elevated water Fe and sulfates can further compromise dietary Cu availability.

The assessment of water quality can be initiated by practical on-farm tools in measuring pH and TDS using battery-powered meters. Commercial and university laboratories offer water analysis testing. Contact the laboratory to determine the method and vessel type for appropriate sample collection and desired testing. If

Table 3
Characterization of 709 forage samples from 23 states relative to mineral content being deficient, marginally deficient, or adequate relative to National Research Council (1996) beef cattle requirements as reported by Mortimer et al (1999)[8,37]

Trace Mineral	Relative to Animal Requirement, % of Samples			Copper Antagonists	
	Deficient	Marginally Deficient	Adequate	Marginal	High
Copper	0.7	66	33.3		
Manganese	0.6	14.1	85.3		
Selenium	43.4	26.1	30.2		
Zinc	33.3	43.7	23.0		
Cu:Mo ratio	15.7	4.8	79.5		
Iron	2.8	0	70.5	18.6	8.0
Sulfur	6.1	22.0	25.5	33.6	12.8
Molybdenum	NA	NA	51.5	40.3	8.2

microbiologic testing is desired samples need to be collected in sterile vessels and submitted within 24 hours of collection. Mineral testing is not as sensitive; however, immediate sampling versus sampling following a period of water flowing can alter results. Many laboratories now provide livestock criteria for evaluating water mineral content (**Fig. 2**).

Dietary Supplements

A range of supplement products can be provided to supply additional minerals; however, under range conditions, free choice mineral products predominate. The use of

	Results	Farm Survey Average	Expected Levels in Drinking	Possible Problem Level for Cattle
pH	6.99	7.0*	6.8 - 7.5	< 5.5 or > 8.5
Nitrate as Nitrogen, ppm	2.52	7.7*	0 - 10	23
Nitrate as NO3, ppm	11.09	33.8*	0 - 44	100
Total Coliform, colonies per 100 ml			< 1	15
E.Coli, Colonies per 100 ml			< 1	10
Hardness, ppm CaCO3	240	208*	0 - 180	
Total Dissolved Solids (TDS), ppm	298	368	0 - 500	3000
Chloride, ppm	18	59	0 - 250	300
Sulfates, ppm	70.9	81	0 - 250	500
Calcium (Ca), ppm	88.1	65	0 - 100	150
Phosphorus (P), ppm	<0.10	0.7	0 - 0.3	0.7
Magnesium (Mg), ppm	4.16	24	0 - 29	100
Potassium (K), ppm	1.40	4	0 - 20	20
Sodium (Na), ppm	6.18	46	0 - 100	300
Iron (Fe), ppm	1.40	0.79	0 - 0.03	0.4 (taste)
Manganese (Mn), ppm	<0.05	0.17	0 - 0.05	0.05 (taste)
Zinc (Zn), ppm	<0.01	0.12	0 - 5	25
Copper (Cu), ppm	<0.01	0.07	0 - 0.6	0.6
Sulfate - Sulfur, ppm		27	0-83	167
Alkalinity		141	0-400	>5000
Molybdenum (Mo), ppm			0-0.068	Not defined
Selenium (Se), ppm				
Boron (Bo)				Not defined

Fig. 2. Example of a laboratory water analysis report. Report provides measured and cautionary mineral concentrations and water properties then provides a color-coded interpretation. Red, level exceeds EPA limits; Yellow, problems likely; Blue, potential problems; and Green, no apparent problems. EPA, Environmental Protection Agency.

inorganic geological compounds is widely used in animal production as mineral supplements supplied with grazing natural forages in beef cattle production. These products may be salt-based or molasses lick tanks in providing mineral sources. Products may contain inorganic, organic, or both mineral sources. Ideally, mineral supplements, due to expense, should only be used when requirements are not met by consumption of forage and water.

Supplements may be commercial or custom formulation. Custom products would be tailored to the mineral needs based on forage and water testing. Commercial products may not properly fit a given ranch's mineral needs potentially under or over supplementing one or more minerals. The key issue with mineral supplementation is the recognized individual variation in intake.[55] Molasses-based lick products suggest a potential intake range and generally are consumed in greater amounts compared with salt-based minerals, though seasonal effects are recognized.[56]

Like forage, any dietary supplement can be appropriately sampled and sent to a laboratory for nutrient content analysis. Collect a representative sample and submit to the laboratory for analysis using wet chemistry methods. Most laboratories will want to know the crude protein content for mineral-fortified products. Be sure to have all the macrominerals determined. This will require special requests for Cl and S.

In lieu of laboratory analysis, commercial products will have an associated feed tag providing pertinent information relative to guaranteed analysis, ingredient listing, and feeding rate. The guaranteed analysis provides limited nutrient composition data based on a state's feed labeling regulations, which may not be sufficient for all trace minerals. The guaranteed analysis will show mineral amounts as primarily minimum content, but Ca and salt will be provided in minimum and maximum values (**Fig. 3**). Ingredients shown will be listed from highest to lowest incorporation rate in the product on an as-fed basis. There may be multiple mineral sources where a combination of inorganic and organic forms may be included. Most importantly one should review the feeding directions indicating the suggested intake rate. Salt content will determine intake, though this will be modified by water availability and salinity and sodium content of forage.

MINERAL PROGRAM STRATEGIES

As indicated, consumption of forage does not completely meet trace mineral needs of the beef cow throughout different life cycle stages. Macro- and micromineral supplementation programs to extensively managed beef cows have consistently shown benefits to cow and calf health and productivity, cow reproduction, and immune function.[57–61] Trace mineral decisions at specific times of the year should focus on supplemental differences that forage grazing cannot meet or provide.[62] Often decisions on mineral supplements are based on what uninformed personnel provide and not based on science or specific needs for the production unit. Using a trained person, veterinarian or nutritionist who understands specific needs, is essential to maximize performance and health. In many instances, professional advice or a custom trace mineral product lowers costs and provides increased health and performance. Mineral supplementation programs should be strategically developed and properly monitored for success (**Box 3**).

Feed costs are the largest single expense for beef cattle production and average ranch mineral-vitamin supplement expense will vary greatly but will usually cost a minimum of $60.00 per cow–calf unit per year for most operations. Most mineral-vitamin supplements have a high cost per ton that can be daunting to the producer; however, the low dietary incorporation rate results in a low dietary component cost. An appropriately formulated specific mineral-vitamin program will be cost-effective in many

Guaranteed Analysis

Calcium, minimum 11.0%
Calcium, maximum 13.0%
Phosphorus, minimum 6.0%
Salt, minimum 20.0%
Salt, maximum 22.0%
Magnesium, minimum 1.0%
Potassium, minimum 2.0%
Copper, minimum.....................................460 ppm
Selenium, minimum ....0.2 ppm
Zinc, minimum ....2300 ppm
Vitamin A, minimum ....100,000 IU/LB

Ingredient Statement

Dicalcium Phosphate, Monocalcium Phosphate, Salt, Manganous Oxide, Zinc Oxide, Ferrous Sulfate, Magnesium Mica, Cane Molasses, Copper Sulfate, Animal Fat, Vitamin A Supplement, D-Activated Animal Sterol (source of Vitamin D_3), Iron Oxide, Animal Fat, Choline Chloride, Biotin, Thiamine Mononitrate, Copper Oxide, Manganese Sulfate, Vitamin E Supplement, Mineral Oil, Sodium Selenite.

FEEDING DIRECTIONS

Feed free-choice at an approximate rate of 4 oz./head/day to beef cattle on pasture. Provide fresh water at all times.

Fig. 3. Example of a mineral supplement feed tag showing only the guaranteed analysis, ingredient listing, and feeding directions. Values of the guaranteed analysis are on an as-fed basis and presented as maximums, minimums, or both depending on the mineral. Ingredient listing is from highest to lowest incorporation rate on an as-fed basis.

ways of reducing health concerns and increasing performance thus decreasing labor for increased production. Custom programs are easily completed by veterinarians as part of value-added service.[63]

Targeted Supplementation

A targeted supplement strategy can be used to better meet cow mineral needs at critical life stages in addition to supplemented mineral. From a mineral nutrient perspective, phosphorus may not be necessary at if pastures have been fertilized or if high-phosphorus byproducts (ie, distiller's grains, wheat middlings) are included in the supplement. Wright has indicated a 1% decline in mineral phosphorus content there is approximately an $11/ton decline in cost.[64] Other minerals that may be in excess in range forage such as Mn, S, or Fe could be removed from the mineral supplement further reducing cost.

Another approach is to target the critical life stages where mineral supplementation will provide the greatest benefit. Based on the research, late gestation through the breeding period would be the most beneficial return.[57–61] One might want to provide minerals above NASEM requirements during these critical times and a lesser amount during other life cycle stages. Wright has provided a table defining trace mineral content relative to 75%, 100%, and 125% of NASEM requirements for products having an expected intake rate between 1 and 4 ounces/head/day (**Table 4**).[64]

Box 3

Organizing a mineral supplementation program for range beef cattle operation

1. *Define Mineral Needs.* Determine mineral needs and formulation accordingly. This varies with geography, age of cattle, and forage and water supplies.
   a. Purchase and design minerals, if possible, on determined forage and water analysis.
   b. Compare prices and products as there will be large variation
   c. Additives can be used in mineral formulations such as sodium monensin and other products.

2. *Evaluate Mineral Intake.* Not all animals of the same size or age consume the same amounts during the same time. Most common problem with mineral deficiencies is intake not necessarily the product used.
   a. Read product label and check to see if intake is what is recommended by the product.
   b. Know that intake variations do often occur with season, rainfall, water supply, and forage species and quality. Be patient for 2 weeks then evaluate.
   c. Intake can be controlled with salt or dried molasses to regulate desired intake. Intake can be increased with molasses-based products compared with salt.

3. *Mineral Feeders.* Enclosed or shaded feeders are recommended to minimize precipitation losses.
   a. Ensure mineral is available. Place a 3 to 4 day's supply of mineral out and check twice weekly and fill as required.
   b. Place mineral for grazing utilization away from water. Place and manage mineral to "rotate" grazing areas.

4. *Program Management and Monitoring.* Must have active management and ongoing monitoring of mineral supplementation.
   a. Assign one person that is in charge of mineral supplementation with a log sheet indicating product, amount used, date, and time, with calculations on intake/period of time to evaluate under or over consumption of the product used.
   b. Initiate animal mineral status assessment process to monitor program outcomes and return on investment.

Frequency and Location of Supplementation

Ideally, balanced diets are consumed on a daily basis; however, with minerals, intermittent feeding is possible assuming that there is hepatic reserve to buffer periods of nonconsumption. Weekly dosing of sheep with the calculated weekly Se intake showed adequate Se status over the entire period.[65] In extensive management systems, providing mineral intermittently is more practical and labor saving. The use of a molasses-based mineral supplement can facilitate more even or desired area grazing.[56] The placement of mineral sources near water sources may induce greater intake.

Methods of Supplementation

Trace minerals are most commonly provided through access to trace mineralized salt products or mineral-fortified energy/protein supplement in beef cattle operations. Both methods require some form of delivering a product to the cow herd. Other targeted options for mineral supplementation are also available for grazing cattle.[62,66]

Free-choice mineral

The principle means by which cattle producers attempt to meet mineral requirements of their grazing herds is through the use of free-choice dietary minerals. Granular form is preferred over blocks. Animals do not have "nutritional knowledge" and only seek out salt or sodium in meeting their needs, thus "cafeteria-style" feeders with separated mineral sources are not appropriate.[67] Salt is used to control intake. Relative to Se, the

Table 4
Suggested trace mineral content (mg/kg [ppm] dry matter) of a salt-based mineral supplement based on expected daily intake (1–4 ounces/day) and meeting 75%, 100%, or 125% of National Research Council requirements for beef cattle

Expected Cow Intake	Trace Mineral					
	Co	Cu	I	Mn	Se	Zn
oz/day	mg/kg or ppm					
75% of NRC Requirement						
1	28.8	2880	144	1152	28.8	8640
2	14.4	1440	72	576	14.4	4320
3	9.6	960	48	384	9.6	2880
4	7.2	720	36	288	7.2	2160
100% of NRC Requirement						
1	38.4	3840	192	15,360	38.4	11,520
2	19.2	1920	96	7680	19.2	5760
3	12.8	1280	64	5120	12.8	3840
4	9.6	960	48	3840	9.6	2880
125% of NRC Requirement						
1	48	4800	240	19,200	48	14,400
2	24	2400	120	9600	24	7200
3	16	1600	80	6400	16	4800
4	12	1200	60	4800	12	3600

Abbreviations: Co, cobalt; Cu, copper; I, iodine; Mn, manganese; Se, selenium; Zn, zinc.
Adapted from Wright, 2003.[64]

Food and Drug Administration allows for 120 ppm Se in free-choice trace mineralized salt assuming an averaged intake of 1.5 ounces/head/day to deliver the maximum 3 mg/head/day supplemental Se. The salt content in these products is 90% to 95%. Many trace mineralized salt products contain 20% to 30% salt or some palatable vehicle accounting for higher expected intake rates. Mineral intakes should be evaluated to determine if the feeding rate is appropriate, otherwise mineral intake may be excessive or deficient (**Box 4**). Individual variation in averaged intake of salt-based products is a significant issue and impacts animal mineral status.[55,62,68]

Box 4
Factors influencing consumption of mineral mixtures

- Soil fertility and forage type
- Season of year
- Available dietary energy and protein
- Individual requirements
- Sodium content of water or forage
- Palatability of mineral mixture
- Availability of fresh minerals
- Physical form of minerals (granular vs block)

Oral bolus

The administration of oral boluses or drenches can deliver a defined mineral amount immediately (drench) or over time (bolus). A slow-release Se bolus had been commercially available in the United States but has since been removed from the market. Australia and New Zealand commonly use drenches or boluses to address their grazing mineral issues.[16,66] Drenching is labor-intensive and not practical in an extensive beef cattle grazing system. Copper oxide wire particle boluses are available for supplementing Cu in grazing systems.[16,66,69] Copper oxide wire particle boluses will release Cu-ions over a period of 6 months. Dosing is based on the interaction of animal size, Cu need, and bolus weight. One author (RJV) has used 20 to 25 g boluses in adult Angus cattle and 10 to 15 g boluses in calves that were found to be Cu-deficient due to elevated forage Mo (>8 mg/kg) content. Excessive bolus administration frequency or size can result in Cu toxicosis, especially in younger calves.[70]

Parenteral

Injectable Se and Cu products have been available for use in beef cattle for some time, though Cu injections often induced injection site necrosis and their use has been limited. More recently, a multi-mineral injectable product has been introduced commercially (MultiMin, MultiMin North America, Ft Collins, CO). The product contains ethylenediaminetetraacetic acid-bound Cu, Mn, and Zn with Na selenite. Studies have shown positive immune function responses, reproductive, and health effects of parenteral mineral injections.[60,62,71] Duration of mineral status following administration was followed out to 30 days.[72,73] Animal mineral status at the time of administration may influence reproductive outcomes.[74] The use of injectable minerals is labor-intensive and may be targeted to known deficiency situations during critical periods. Oral mineral supplementation should remain the primary mode of mineral supplementation.

Biofortification of forage

Soil fertilization with the intent to increase plant mineral content is the process of biofortification. This process is being used in many countries with many trace minerals. Studies using Se-fertilization to increase forage Se content have shown very positive responses in maintaining adequate Se status over the grazing period, improved animal health, and augmented immune function.[75–77] The positive response to Se-enriched forage compared with inorganic Se supplementation is related to the organic form (eg, selenomethionine, selenocysteine) in Se-fertilized forage. Unfortunately, the use of Se fertilization is only legal in the state of Oregon within the United States at present.

TRACE MINERAL ASSESSMENT

Assessing trace mineral status of a beef herd can be accomplished by determining estimated intake from all consumed sources (eg, forage, water, and supplements) and compared with defined nutrient requirements accounting for the recognized mitigating factors influencing mineral availability. A second method is through determination of the animal's trace mineral status. Depending on the trace mineral, serum or liver samples can be used to determine trace mineral concentration and compared with laboratory reference values.[78]

Blood Mineral Analysis

The collection of blood is a reasonably simple sampling method for beef cattle. Samples can be collected whenever cattle are being restrained and handled. The challenge is that serum or plasma trace mineral concentrations are not sufficiently adequate to interpret mineral status, except for Se.[78–80] Even with Se, serum concentration can be artificially elevated with hemolysis in the sample, thus some suggest whole blood Se concentration as a preferred measurement.[81] Individual blood mineral concentrations are not accurate in assessing mineral nutritive state due to the large variation among individuals. The collection of multiple samples to account for the individual variation and assess the "herd" effect directed through the nutrition program can be used to assess a herd's nutritional program.[79,80] Sampling between 10 and 15 individuals can provide a better perspective of the herd nutritional program.[79,80] The downside of this approach is the cost of performing the trace mineral analysis.

Liver Mineral Analysis

The liver is considered the primary storage site for most trace minerals, except for I. The determination of hepatic mineral concentrations is considered the best method for assessing mineral nutritive status of the animal and herd collectively.[78] With newer methodologies for mineral analysis, a smaller biopsy instrument can be used to collect an appropriate liver biopsy sample for analysis. This reduces the potential complications for the biopsy procedure compared with the past methods.[82] Even so, there still remains producer apprehension in having liver biopsies performed as part of mineral assessment diagnostics.

Hair Mineral Analysis

Often producers are presented with information suggesting their mineral program can be evaluated through mineral analysis of hair. Hair sampling is challenging as there is significant mineral contamination from soil, detergents, seasonal hair growth, and other factors.[83,84] Hair may be an indicator of toxic mineral exposure such as with Se. Hair mineral analysis coupled with other methods may be a reasonable use.[83,85]

SUMMARY

Interaction between trace mineral requirements and bovine production is very complex and not fully understood with many factors affecting trace mineral supplementation response as mineral concentration, physiology of the bovine animal, presence or absence of trace mineral antagonists, soil, water, or environmental factors, and other complex factors of the animal including performance goals, stress, and host tissue metabolism. There is no question as beef cattle genetics improve in beef cattle production the need for optimal supplemental mineral nutrition will be challenged. Mineral supplementation has been shown to be necessary in range beef cattle production as forage does not inadequately supply all trace minerals and availability may be compromised by common antagonists in forage and water. Controlled studies support the use of supplementation, especially during last gestation through breeding as evidenced by improved cow and calf health and performance. Supplying a free-choice trace mineralized salt product appropriate for the determined needs of a given ranch's situation is the most economic and practical approach.

CLINICS CARE POINTS

- Mineral intake from forage and water sources as well as the presence of antagonistic agents is the basis of determining supplemental mineral needs for the cattle class, age, and production goals of the ranch.
- In most cases, an investment in designing a custom product that fits specific ranch needs is cost-effective after the purchase of only two tons of product. The use of an independent nutritionist for a more detailed formulation is desirable.

- Target mineral supplementation during late gestation through early lactation to ensure adequate trace mineral transfer to fetus and colostrum to ensure calf health and immune function.
- Average mineral supplement intake needs to be evaluated to ensure appropriate mineral supply given recognized individual variation.
- Animal mineral status assessment using serum and liver biopsy sample mineral concentrations is needed to ensure the mineral program is achieving desired results.

DISCLOSURES

There is no commercial or financial conflicts in this article by the author. Grant funding received from Pennsylvania Department of Agriculture, United States, American Dairy Goat Association, United States, Zoetis, United States.

REFERENCES

1. Leng R. Factors affecting the utilization of 'poor-quality'forages by ruminants particularly under tropical conditions. Nutr Res Rev 1990;3:277–303.
2. Martinez A, Church D. Effect of various mineral elements on in vitro rumen cellulose digestion. J Anim Sci 1970;31:982–90.
3. National Academies of Sciences Engineering and Medicine (NASEM). Nutrient requirements of beef cattle. 8th Revised Edition. Washington, DC: The National Academies Press; 2016.
4. Suttle NF. Problems in the diagnosis and anticipation of trace element deficiencies in grazing livestock. Vet Rec 1986;119:148–52.
5. Suttle NF. Mineral nutrition of livestock. 4th edition. Oxfordshire, UK: CABI International; 2010.
6. National Research Council (NRC). Nutrient requirements of domestic animals. 4. Nutrient requirements of beef cattle. Washington, DC: National Academies Press; 1958.
7. National Research Council (NRC). Nutrient requirements of beef cattle. 5th revised edition. Washington, DC: National Academies Press; 1984.
8. National Research Council (NRC). Nutrient requirements of beef cattle. 7th revised edition. Washington, DC: National Academies Press; 1996.
9. National Research Council (NRC). Nutrient requirements of beef cattle: 7th revised edition: update 2000. Washington, DC: National Academies Press; 2000.
10. Swecker T. Trace mineral feeding and assessment. Vet Clinics NA: Food Anim Pract 2023;39(3).
11. McDowell LR. Minerals in animal and human nutrition. San Diego, CA: Academic Press Inc; 1992.
12. Buchweitz JP, Scheffler R, Puschner B. Trace mineral toxicosis in ruminants. Vet Clinics NA: Food Anim Pract 2023;39(3).
13. National Research Council (NRC). Selenium in nutrition: revised edition. Washington, DC: National Academies Press; 1983.
14. James L, Panter K, Mayland H, et al. Selenium poisoning in livestock: a review and progress. Selenium in Agriculture and the Environment 1989;23:123–31.
15. O'Toole D, Raisbeck M, Case JC, et al. Selenium-induced "blind staggers" and related myths. A commentary on the extent of historical livestock losses attributed to selenosis on western US rangelands. Vet Pathol 1996;33:109–16.

16. Lee J, Masters D, Judson G, et al. Current issues in trace element nutrition of grazing livestock in Australia and New Zealand. Aust J Agric Res 1999;50: 1341–64.

17. Olson KC. Management of mineral supplementation programs for cow-calf operations. Vet Clin North Am Food Anim Pract 2007;23:69–90.

18. Bittar JH, Palomares RA. A research-based summary on trace minerals for cattle. VM245. Gainesville, Fl: University of Florida; 2021. https://doi.org/10.32473/edis-VM245-2021.

19. Wikse S. The relationship of trace element deficiencies to infectious diseases of beef calves. Texas A&M University: Texas Beef Short Course; 1992.

20. Spears JW. Micronutrients and Immune Function in Cattle. Proc Nutr Soc 2000; 59:587–94.

21. Wright CL, Corah LR, Stokka G, et al. Effects of pre-weaning vitamin E, selenium, and copper supplementation on the performance, acute phase protein concentration, and immune function of stressed beef calves. Prof Anim Sci 2000;16: 111–20.

22. Toombs RE, Wikse SE, Kasari TR. The incidence, causes, and financial impact of perinatal mortality in North American beef herds. Vet Clin North Am Food Anim Pract 1994;10:137–46.

23. Capper JL. The environmental impact of beef production in the United States: 1977 compared with 2007. J Anim Sci 2011;89:4249–61.

24. Gooneratne S, Christensen D, Bailey J, et al. Effects of dietary copper, molybdenum and sulfur on biliary copper and zinc excretion in Simmental and Angus cattle. Can J Anim Sci 1994;74:315–25.

25. Ward J, Spears J, Gengelbach G. Differences in copper status and copper metabolism among Angus, Simmental, and Charolais cattle. J Anim Sci 1995;73: 571–7.

26. Fry R, Spears J, Lloyd K, et al. Effect of dietary copper and breed on gene products involved in copper acquisition, distribution, and use in Angus and Simmental cows and fetuses. J Anim Sci 2013;91:861–71.

27. Sager RB, Yeoman CJ, Duff GC. Cobalt supplementation in pre-weaned beef calves affects humoral immune response and feedlot health. In: Proc western section25-27. San Angelo, TX: American Society of Animal Science; 2014. p. 162–5.

28. Goff JP. Invited review: Mineral absorption mechanisms, mineral interactions that affect acid-base and antioxidant status, and diet considerations to improve mineral status. J Dairy Sci 2018;101:2763–813.

29. Spears JW. Trace mineral bioavailability in ruminants. J Nutr 2003;133:1506S–9S.

30. Hansen SL, Trakooljul N, Liu HC, et al. Proteins involved in iron metabolism in beef cattle are affected by copper deficiency in combination with high dietary manganese, but not by copper deficiency alone. J Anim Sci 2010;88:275–83.

31. Gould L, Kendall NR. Role of the rumen in copper and thiomolybdate absorption. Nutr Res Rev 2011;24:176–82.

32. Smith B, Wright H. Copper: Molybdenum interaction: Effect of dietary molybdenum on the binding of copper to plasma proteins in sheep. J Comp Path 1975; 85:299–305.

33. Suttle N. The interactions between copper, molybdenum, and sulphur in ruminant nutrition. Annu Rev Nutr 1991;11:121–40.

34. Suttle NF. Recent studies of the copper-molybdenum antagonism. Proc Nutr Soc 1974;33:299–305.

35. Darch T, McGrath SP, Lee MRF, et al. The mineral composition of wild-type and cultivated varieties of pasture species. Agronomy 2020;10.
36. Miltimore J, Mason J. Copper to molybdenum ratio and molybdenum and copper concentrations in ruminant feeds. Can J Anim Sci 1971;51:193–200.
37. Mortimer R, Dargatz D, Corah L. Forage analyses from cow-calf herds in 23 states in: USDA:APHIS:vs. Fort Collins, CO: enters for Epidemiology and Animal Health; 1999. p. 31.
38. Ward GM. Molybdenum toxicity and hypocuprosis in ruminants: a review. J Anim Sci 1978;46:1078–85.
39. Spears J. Advancements in ruminant trace mineral nutrition. In: Proc cornell nutrition Conference for feed manufacturers. NY: East Syracuse; 2013. p. 11–7.
40. Beutler KT, Pankewycz O, Brautigan DL. Equivalent uptake of organic and inorganic zinc by monkey kidney fibroblasts, human intestinal epithelial cells, or perfused mouse intestine. Biol Trace Elem Res 1998;61:19–31.
41. Knowles SO, Grace N, Wurms K, et al. Significance of Amount and Form of Dietary Selenium on Blood, Milk, and Casein Selenium Concentrations in Grazing Cows. J Dairy Sci 1999;82:429–37.
42. Pehrson B, Ortman K, Madjid N, et al. The Influence of Dietary Selenium as Selenium Yeast or Sodium Selenite on the Concentration of Selenium in the Milk of Suckler Cows and on the Selenium Status of Their Calves. J Anim Sci 1999; 77:3371–6.
43. Spears JW. Organic trace minerals in ruminant nutrition. Anim Feed Sci Technol 1996;58:151–63.
44. Spears JW. Evaluation of trace mineral sources. Vet Clinics NA: Food Anim Pract 2023;39(3).
45. Van Saun RJ. Feed supplements: microminerals and organic-chelated minerals. In: McSweeney PLH, McNamara JP, editors. Encyclopedia of dairy sciences. 3rd edition. Amsterdam, Netherlands: Elsevier Academic Press; 2021. p. 527–39.
46. Miles RD, Henry PR. Relative trace mineral bioavailability. Ciencia Anim Bras 2000;1:73–93.
47. Whitehead DC. Nutrient elements in grassland: soil-plant-animal relationships. Wallingford, Oxon, UK: CABI Publishing; 2000.
48. McBride MB. Molybdenum and Copper Uptake by Forage Grasses and Legumes Grown on a Metal-Contaminated Sludge Site. Commun Soil Sci Plant Anal 2007; 36:2489–501.
49. Jones G, Wade NS, Baker JP, et al. Use of near infrared reflectance spectroscopy in forage testing. J Dairy Sci 1987;70:1086–91.
50. Socha MT, Ensley S, Tomlinson DJ, et al. Variability of water composition and potential impact on animal performance. In: Proc Intermountain Nutrition Conference 2003; Salt Lake City, UT, p. 85-96.
51. Morgan SE. Water quality for cattle. Vet Clin North Am Food Anim Pract 2011; 27(2):285–95.
52. Bagley CV, Amacher JK, Poe KF. Analysis of water quality for livestock. AH/Beef 1997;28:1.
53. Swistock B. Interpreting drinking water tests for dairy cows. 2012. Available at www.extension.psu.edu; Accessed August 1, 2023.
54. Patterson T, Johnson P. Effects of water quality on beef cattle. In: The Range Beef Cow Symposium XVIII 2003; Mitchell, NB, Dec 9-11, 8 pp.
55. Tait R, Fisher L. Variability in individual animal's intake of minerals offered free-choice to grazing ruminants. Anim Feed Sci Technol 1996;62:69–76.

56. Aubel NA, Jaeger JR, Drouillard JS, et al. Effects of mineral-supplement delivery system on frequency, duration, and timing of supplement use by beef cows grazing topographically rugged, native rangeland in the Kansas Flint Hills. J Anim Sci 2011;89:3699–706.

57. Harvey KM, Cooke RF, Marques RDS. Supplementing Trace Minerals to Beef Cows during Gestation to Enhance Productive and Health Responses of the Offspring. Animals (Basel) 2021;11:1159.

58. Hurlbert JL, Baumgaertner F, McCarthy KL, et al. Effects of feeding a vitamin and mineral supplement to cow-calf pairs grazing native range. Transl Anim Sci 2023; 7:txad077.

59. Marques RS, Cooke RF, Rodrigues MC, et al. Effects of organic or inorganic cobalt, copper, manganese, and zinc supplementation to late-gestating beef cows on productive and physiological responses of the offspring. J Anim Sci 2016;94: 1215–26.

60. Palomares RA. Trace Minerals Supplementation with Great Impact on Beef Cattle Immunity and Health. Animals (Basel) 2022;12:2839.

61. Stanton T, Whittier J, Geary T, et al. Effects of trace mineral supplementation on cow-calf performance, reproduction, and immune function. Prof Anim Sci 2000; 16:121–7.

62. Arthington JD, Ranches J. Trace Mineral Nutrition of Grazing Beef Cattle. Animals (Basel) 2021;11:2767.

63. Larson RL. Calculating Supplementation Requirements for Trace Mineral Deficiency. Agri Pract 1996;17:6–10.

64. Wright CL. Making $ense of Mineral Supplementation. In: The Range Beef Cow Symposium XVIII 2003; Mitchell, NB, Dec 9-11, p. 64-74.

65. Hall JA, Van Saun RJ, Bobe G, et al. Organic and inorganic selenium: I. Oral bioavailability in ewes. J Anim Sci 2012;90:568–76.

66. Grace ND, Knowles SO. Trace element supplementation of livestock in New Zealand: Meeting the challenges of free-range grazing systems. Vet Med Int 2012; 2012:639472.

67. Muller LD, Schaffer LV, Ham LC, et al. Cafeteria style free-choice mineral feeder for lactating dairy cows. J Dairy Sci 1977;60:1574–82.

68. Cockwill C, McAllister T, Olson M, et al. Individual intake of mineral and molasses supplements by cows, heifers and calves. Can J Anim Sci 2000;80:681–90.

69. Arthington JD. Effects of copper oxide bolus administration or high-level copper supplementation on forage utilization and copper status in beef cattle. J Anim Sci 2005;83:2894–900.

70. Steffen DJ, Carlson MP, Casper HH. Copper toxicosis in suckling beef calves with improper administration of copper oxid boluses. J Vet Diagn Invest 1997;9:443–6.

71. Palomares RA, Hurley DJ, Bittar JH, et al. Effects of injectable trace minerals on humoral and cell-mediated immune responses to Bovine viral diarrhea virus, Bovine herpes virus 1 and Bovine respiratory syncytial virus following administration of a modified-live virus vaccine in dairy calves. Vet Immunol Immunopathol 2016;178:88–98.

72. Genther ON, Hansen SL. A multielement trace mineral injection improves liver copper and selenium concentrations and manganese superoxide dismutase activity in beef steers. J Anim Sci 2014;92:695–704.

73. Pogge DJ, Richter EL, Drewnoski ME, et al. Mineral concentrations of plasma and liver after injection with a trace mineral complex differ among Angus and Simmental cattle. J Anim Sci 2012;90:2692–8.

74. Willmore CJ, Hall JB, Drewnoski ME. Effect of a Trace Mineral Injection on Performance and Trace Mineral Status of Beef Cows and Calves. Animals (Basel) 2021;11.
75. Hall JA, Bobe G, Hunter JK, et al. Effect of feeding selenium-fertilized alfalfa hay on performance of weaned beef calves. PLoS One 2013;8:e58188.
76. Ranches J, Vendramini JMB, Arthington JD. Effects of selenium biofortification of hayfields on measures of selenium status in cows and calves consuming these forages. J Anim Sci 2017;95.
77. Wallace LG, Bobe G, Vorachek WR, et al. Effects of feeding pregnant beef cows selenium-enriched alfalfa hay on selenium status and antibody titers in their newborn calves. J Anim Sci 2017;95.
78. Ensley S. Evaluating Mineral Status in Ruminant Livestock. Vet Clin North Am Food Anim Pract 2020;36:525–46.
79. Herdt TH, Hoff B. The use of blood analysis to evaluate trace mineral status in ruminant livestock. Vet Clin North Am Food Anim Pract 2011;27:255–83.
80. Herdt TH, Rumbeiha W, Braselton WE. The Use of Blood Analyses to Evaluate Mineral Status in Livestock. Vet Clin North Am Food Anim Pract 2000;16:423–44.
81. Maas J, Peauroi JR, Tonjes T, et al. Intramuscular Selenium Administration in Selenium-Deficient Cattle. J Vet Intern Med 1993;7:342–8.
82. Herdt TH. Liver Biopsy Procedure in Cattle. 2021; Available at: https://cvm.msu.edu/vdl/laboratory-sections/nutrition/mineral-and-vitamin-testing-sample-collection-and-handling/liver-biopsy-procedure-in-cattle. Accessed July 20, 2023.
83. Combs D. Hair analysis as an indicator of mineral status of livestock. J Anim Sci 1987;65:1753–8.
84. Combs D, Goodrich R, Meiske J. Mineral concentrations in hair as indicators of mineral status: a review. J Anim Sci 1982;54:391–8.
85. Keating J. Hair analysis in cattle as an index of mineral status. Ir Vet J 1960; 14:74–8.

Vitamin and Trace Element Nutrition of Stocker Cattle on Small Grain and Winter Annual Pastures

Paul A. Beck, MS, PhD, MBA[a],*, Jeffery O. Hall, DVM, PhD[b,1]

KEYWORDS

- Small grain forages • Trace minerals • Liver analysis • Beef cattle

KEY POINTS

- There is considerable variation in the mineral composition of small grain forages, depending on management, growth conditions, and soil mineral content.
- Small grain forages can be deficient in macrominerals; such as calcium and magnesium, as well as trace minerals, in particular copper, zinc, and selenium.
- Testing forages provide information helpful for formulating mineral supplements to address deficiencies.
- Antagonists such as molybdenum and sulfur must be considered when formulating mineral supplements.
- Increased gains in cattle grazing small grain forages have been demonstrated when proper mineral supplements are provided.

INTRODUCTION

Wheat and other small grain forages are important forage resources for cattle producers in the Southern Great Plains, the Western Gulf Coastal Plains of the Southeastern US, and into the mid-South region, where cool season perennial grass species do not persist. Winter wheat pasture is an economically important resource for crop producers in the Southern Great Plains region including much of central and western Oklahoma, southern Kansas, the Texas and Oklahoma Panhandles, and north central Texas where wheat and other small grain species are used in a "dual purpose" production system.[1,2] Growing calves or cow calf pairs graze wheat

[a] Department of Animal and Food Sciences, Oklahoma State University, 4343 South Highway 23, Wellsville, UT 84339, USA; [b] Huvepharma Inc., 525 Westpark Drive, Suite 230, Peachtree City, GA 30269, USA
[1] Present address: 4343 South Highway 23, Wellsville, UT 84339.
* Corresponding author.
E-mail address: paul.beck@okstate.edu

Vet Clin Food Anim 39 (2023) 491–504
https://doi.org/10.1016/j.cvfa.2023.05.005
vetfood.theclinics.com

fields during the fall and winter and wheat grain can be harvested with little loss in yield if cattle are removed prior to the first hollow stem developmental stage of the wheat plant in the late winter or early spring.[1,2] Income thus can come from both harvested grain and the increased value of weight gain to growing cattle grazed on wheat pastures.

In the Gulf Coastal Plains and Southeastern US, wheat and other small grains are often "interseeded" or planted into sod forming introduced grass pastures such as bermudagrass or bahiagrass close to or shortly after summer grasses have gone dormant in the fall.[3–5] This system extends the grazing season beyond the production of the predominantly warm-season perennial forage base with high-quality forages.

Small grain forages are high in crude protein (17%–35% of DM) and are highly digestible (up to 85% *in vitro* organic matter degradability), which is adequate for potential average daily gains in excess of 2.5 pounds per day.[6] However, these performance levels are often not achieved in practice, where growth performance is impacted by forage availability, seasonal bloat outbreaks, as well as nutritional deficiencies and imbalances.[7] Multiple macro and trace minerals are among the key nutritional deficiencies and nutrient imbalances implicated in performance and health of beef cattle consuming small grain forages.[7]

In this review, we discuss the mineral content and subsequent deficiencies, imbalances, and interactions found in wheat and small grain pastures, response to supplementation, and determining mineral status in vivo. Although the dominant theme of this article is trace mineral nutrition, there are significant macromineral issues in cattle grazing small grain forages that warrant discussion.

Mineral Content of Small Grain Pastures

Mineral analysis of fresh wheat forage from the Dairy One Forage Laboratory Feed Composition Library[8] in the accumulated years from 2004 to 2022 is presented in **Table 1**. In general, small grain pastures can be considered to be very low in Ca (see **Table 1**). The Dairy One Feed Composition Library reported average Ca at

Table 1
Macro (% of DM) and trace mineral (mg/kg of DM) content of fresh wheat forage analyzed at the dairy one forage laboratory for years from 2004 to 2022

Item	NASEM Requirement[b]	Dairy One[a]			
		Average	N	Standard Deviation	Range
Ca, %	0.73	0.38	1984	0.181	0.19–0.55
P, %	0.35	0.31	1989	0.095	0.22–0.41
Mg, %	0.10	0.17	1897	0.069	0.10–0.24
K, %	0.60	2.54	1902	0.971	1.57–3.52
S, %	0.15	0.20	1651	0.133	0.13–0.27
Fe, mg/kg	50	509	643	577.3	0–1086
Cu, mg/kg	10.0	8.4	641	3.70	4.8–12.2
Mn, mg/kg	20.0	58.5	641	54.17	4.4–113.7
Mo, mg/kg	-	1.8	634	2.05	0–3.9
Zn, mg/kg	30.0	30.3	644	12.39	17.9–42.7

[a] Dairy One Forage Laboratory–Feed Composition Library, Dairy One, 2023.(8).
[b] National Academies of Science, Engineering and Medicine, 2016 Beef Cattle Nutrient Requirements Model. Based on a Hereford × Angus growing steer weighing 550 pounds grazing wheat pasture with 25% crude protein and 85% digestibility (NASEM, 2016).

0.38% with a range from 0.19% to 0.55% juxtaposed with a requirement of 0.73% of dietary DM.[9] This compares reasonably well with research compiled by Beck and Reuter (2022)[7] from 3 published experiments in northern Arkansas, central Oklahoma, and northwest Oklahoma with average Ca of 0.38 ($\pm$0.091) % of DM.[7] These values are characteristic of small grains forages in general. Therefore, Ca is the macromineral of primary concern in many wheat pasture-grazing situations.[9]

The average P analysis of wheat forage in this database (Dairy One, 2023)[8] indicates a marginal deficiency in P with sufficient Mg. The high K content of wheat forage is problematic because K interferes with Mg absorption in the gastrointestinal tract. Grass tetany is not considered a problem for growing cattle grazing small grain pastures, but is an issue with mature cows. Grass tetany in mature cows is caused by low blood Mg levels that can result from either low Mg intake or poor absorption. It is commonly a problem in nursing cows grazing small grain pastures in the spring[10] due to Mg excretion in the milk and reduced the resorption of Mg from the bone in mature cows compared with younger cows or growing calves. Grass tetany potential is based on the ratio of the molecular weight of K to the molecular weights of Ca and Mg.[11] This is calculated by (K/39)/([Ca/20] + [Mg/12.1]) and should be < 2.2. This equation was developed for lactating cows and has not been tested for use in growing cattle.

High dietary N has been associated with lower serum Mg and increased incidence of grass tetany as well.[12] Also, feeding high levels of P with low Ca levels has likewise been shown to reduce Mg absorption and serum concentration,[12] thus small grain pastures with their low Ca and higher P content are especially problematic in Mg nutrition.

While it is a common misconception that growing cattle on small grain pasture can suffer from grass tetany, Mg deficiency is a real potential issue for growing cattle grazing small grain forages. Even though grass tetany is not an issue with young growing cattle, the complex interactions of high N, K, and P along with low Ca in small grain forages shows that Mg deficiency may be problematic even though a laboratory analysis indicates adequacy.[7] Beck and Reuter (2022)[7] recommended that Mg be supplied in mineral supplements to offset these mineral interactions.

There are indications that the mineral status associated with wheat pasture may also affect bloat, which is often an acute issue in rapidly growing wheat pasture in the early spring. Pastures with mineral profiles indicating grass tetany potential have also been linked to severe bloat outbreaks on pasture.10 Wheat pasture bloat is often associated with high levels of soluble proteins in pastures,[10,13] but it is thought that this issue may be exacerbated by mineral deficiencies and interactions. Calcium and Mg have roles in muscle contraction; thus deficiencies could compromise ruminal motility and contribute to bloat.

Trace Minerals

From the database presented in **Table 1**, Mn would be considered adequate, Fe in excess, Zn could be considered marginal, and Cu deficient. There is considerable variation in the mineral composition of small grain forages, depending on management, growth conditions, and soil mineral content. For example, small grain forages grown on Coastal Plain soils are notably low in Cu (<10 mg/kg of forage DM) and other trace minerals, but in contrast often contains high concentrations of Mo and S.[14,15] The low concentration of trace minerals in winter-annual grasses is likely a result of shallow root systems caused by frequent rainfalls during winter months. The soils associated with Coastal Plain soils are noted for their low organic matter, base saturation, and low cation exchange capacity.[16] As plants grow, hydrogen ions are released from root hairs and these hydrogen ions force cations, such as Cu, to be released into soil water and then assimilated with the absorptive surfaces of the roots. However, when soils have a low cation exchange capacity and base saturation, cations are not as efficiently released from the soil's exchange complex, resulting in plant tissue low in the mineral in question.[16]

To evaluate the ability of winter annual pasture to supply Cu, Zn, and Se, 8 Angus sired calves (4 steers and 4 heifers; BW = 157 ± 9.5 kg) were allowed to graze winter annual pasture for 169 d without trace mineral supplementation from December 4 to May 21, 2003.[17] Blood and plasma were collected on approximately 35-day intervals for whole blood Se and plasma Zn and Cu analysis and muscle biopsies were collected on day 0 and 169 from the gluteus maximus for Cu, Se, and Zn determination. The macro and trace mineral concentrations averaged throughout the grazing period are presented in **Table 2**. Mineral concentrations were within the ranges reported by Dairy One labs[8] (see **Table 1**). The pastures grazed in this experiment would be considered adequate in P, Mg S, Mn, and Zn; but deficient in Ca, Se, and Cu. Calves gained over 1.06 kg/d without TM supplementation even though whole blood Se and plasma Cu concentrations decreased 83% and 28%, respectively, in a quadratic ($P < .01$) fashion (Se = 174, 108, 78, 52, 32, and 29 ng/mL and Cu = 0.99, 0.74, 0.72, 0.63, 0.67, and 0.71 µg/mL for day 0, 36, 70, 98, 140, and 169, respectively). Whole blood Se was suggested to be marginal (60–150 ng Se/mL) for optimal GSH-Px activity and immune function[18] on day 36 and 70. From day 98 through the end of the grazing period whole blood Se concentrations indicate deficiency.[18] Concentrations of Cu in blood serum would be considered marginal by the Netherlands Committee on Mineral Nutrition (1973),[19] but are slightly higher than the marginal band (0.19–0.57 mg Cu L–1) suggested by Underwood and Suttle (1999).[20] Although serum Cu concentrations are correlated with liver Cu, these associations are not strong enough to predict actual Cu status by serum concentrations.[21]

Steers grazing wheat pastures in the western Gulf Coastal Plains region of Arkansas were supplemented for 29 days before shipping to a High Plains feedyard with grain-

Table 2
Macro (% of DM) and Trace Mineral (mg/kg of DM) Content of Small Grain and Other Winter Annual Pastures from Locations in the Gulf Coastal Plain (GCP), Southeastern US (SE), and Southern Great Plains region in Central Oklahoma (COK) and northwest Oklahoma (NWOK)

Item	#1	#2	#3	#4	#5
Citation	Gunter, et al,[17] 2006	Beck, et al,[22] 2002	Gunter, et al,[31] 2003	Fieser, et al,[33] 2007	Gunter and Combs,[34] 2019
Location	GCP	GCP	GCP	COK	NWOK
Ca	0.39	0.49	0.45	0.47	0.31
P	0.57	0.29	0.50	0.19	0.20
Mg	0.22	0.17	0.17	0.28	0.14
K	3.43	1.55	-	2.36	1.75
S	0.23	0.21	0.29	0.28	0.21
Fe	262	630	90	721	858
Se	0.05	-	0.11	-	0.09
Cu	6.9	10.0	6	6.8	4.2
Mn	360	194	156	282	149
Mo	-	2.0	-	-	0.47
Zn	34.5	30.0	25.0	25.0	16.2

based supplements formulated to provide 21 mg/kg supplemental Cu from CuSO4 or an additional 150 mg/kg Cu as Cu proteinate (Bioplex Cu, Alltech, Inc.) for a total of 171 mg/kg of supplemental Cu.[22] The concentration of minerals in the forage samples collected from the winter annual pastures (see **Table 2**) was 0.49% Ca, 0.29% P, 0.17% Mg, 1.55% K, 0.21% S, 630 mg/kg Fe, 30 mg/kg Zn, 10 mg/kg Cu, 194 mg/kg Mn, and 2.0 mg/kg Mo (DM basis). There are some important items to note about the forage analysis. Zinc and Cu concentrations (30 and 10 ppm, respectively) would be considered adequate for growing livestock,[9,23] but the Mo concentration was relatively high (2 ppm). Molybdenum has been shown to inhibit the absorption of Cu and decrease the growth rate of beef calves.[24–27] Ratios of Cu:Mo in diets less than 2:1 result in a "conditioned" Cu deficiency.[28] This "conditioned" Cu deficiency on Coastal Plain soils is probably a result of management for highly productive pasture. The pH of these inherently acidic soils[29] must be increased by liming for maximum production which in turn decreases plant Cu uptake and increases Mo absorption.[30] Steers supplemented with additional Cu proteinate for 29 days had 0.1 kg/d increased average daily gains on wheat pasture compared to cattle fed the control supplement. This advantage was also maintained through the feedlot receiving period. Serum Cu concentration on d 0 averaged 0.57 mg/L and did not differ between treatments. On d 29 of grazing, the serum Cu concentration had increased 12.4% compared to d 0, but still did not differ between Cu treatments, indicating that these steers could have benefited from even greater levels or a longer period of Cu supplementation. During feedlot receiving, Cu proteinate supplementation increased serum Cu concentration by 6.8% by day d 42, but did not impact gain performance. Thus, the inclusion of Cu proteinate was able to offset the conditioned Cu deficiency caused by mineral interactions.

Beef cows in the Gulf Coastal Plains region of southwest Arkansas grazed bermudagrass-base pastures for 2 years to determine the effects of supplemental Se and the source of Se on performance and blood measurements.[31] During the winter, each group of cows had ad libitum access to bermudagrass/dallisgrass hay plus they were allowed limited access (1–4 d/wk) to a 2.4-ha winter-annual paddock planted in half the pasture. Cows had ad libitum access to 1 of 3 free-choice minerals: (1) no supplemental Se, (2) 26 mg of supplemental Se from sodium selenite/kg, and (3) 26 mg of supplemental Se from seleno-yeast/kg (designed intake = 113 g/cow daily). The bermudagrass/dallisgrass hay fed during the winter averaged (DM basis) 11% CP and 56% TDN over the 2-yr period. Mineral analysis from the small grain forage used as a supplement for cows is shown in **Table 2**. Calcium, P, Mg, S, Mn, and Fe concentrations in both hay and winter-annual pasture samples exceeded the NASEM (2016) requirements.[9] Sulfur is a known antagonist to trace minerals which can exacerbate the deficient Cu and Zn observed in this study. Neither Se supplementation or source of Se significantly affected cow or calf performance. At the beginning of the calving and breeding seasons cows supplemented with Se had greater whole blood Se and glutathione peroxidase activity than controls, and feeding the selenized yeast had greater whole blood Se than cows fed sodium selenite, but glutathione peroxidase activity did not differ between sources. Supplementing Se to cows increased their calves' whole blood Se at birth and near peak lactation compared with controls. Also, feeding selenized yeast to cows increased blood Se and glutathione peroxidase activity of their calves compared with calves from dams supplemented with sodium selenite. Calves from cows fed supplements without Se were still considered to be Se deficient based on whole blood and glutathione peroxidase activity analysis, which was increased by Se supplementation.[32] Feeding selenized yeast further increased Se status compared with sodium selenite. In vitro lymphocyte proliferation was not statistically different in unstimulated cultures or cultures stimulated with pokeweed mitogen, concanavalin A, or phytohemagglutinin, but macrophage phagocytosis was increased with selenized yeast compared with control or sodium selenite. In vivo cell-mediated immunity was also estimated by the swelling reaction to an intradermal phytohemagglutinin injection. Swelling response tended to increase with Se supplementation compared with controls, indicating Se deficiency impaired the immune system's ability to respond to mitogens.

The effects of the mineral supplementation of steers grazing wheat pasture have been reported in experiments from 2 locations in Oklahoma (Oklahoma State University) Wheat Pasture Research Unit [MPRU] reported by Fieser and colleagues (2007)[33] and USDA ARS Southern Plains Range Research Station [SPRRS] reported by Gunter and Combs (2019)[34] and 1 location in Arkansas (University of Arkansas Livestock and Forestry Research Station [UA LFRS] reported by Beck and colleagues [2021][35]). In these experiments, a balanced, complete mineral designed to match the deficiencies for growing calves grazing wheat pasture was offered in comparison to plain white salt (LFRS) or no supplemental mineral (MWPRU and SPRRS). The reported mineral supplement composition fed in these experiments is presented in **Table 3**. Mineral supplements contained greater Ca than P in order to correct the Ca deficiency and unbalanced Ca:P ratio (see **Table 1**), and also contained low levels of K. Magnesium levels in the mineral supplements were designed specifically for wheat pasture stocker calves (ie, lower Mg than mineral supplements designed for beef cows grazing pastures with high grass tetany potential). Minerals were designed for a target intake of 4 oz/day, and actual mineral intakes ranged from 107% to 164% of the target.

The gain responses of growing steers in these experiments are presented in **Fig. 1**. Fieser and co-workers (2007)33 found that providing a balanced mineral supplement did not significantly increase daily gains when performance was limited to 0.5 kg/day on wheat pasture in yr 1 (MWPRU, yr 1; see **Fig. 1**). Yet, growing steers fed a non-medicated mineral gained 0.22 kg more per day than steers receiving no supplement when forage resources were adequate for gains in excess of 0.91 kg/d (MWPRU, yr 2; see **Fig. 1**). Gunter and Combs (2019)34 showed that gains of calves provided a balanced mineral supplement were 20% (SPRRS, Fall; see **Fig. 1**) to 43% (SPRRS, Spring; see **Fig. 1**) greater than cattle that were provided no mineral supplement.

Table 3
Reported composition of mineral supplements offered to growing calves grazing wheat pasture

Citation	Fieser et al,[33] 2007 Year 1	Fieser et al,[33] 2007 Year 2	Gunter and Combs,[34] 2019	Beck et al,[35] 2021
Study Site	MWPRU	MWPRU	SPRRS	UA LFRS
Target intake, oz/day	4.0	4.0	4.0	4.0
Actual intake, oz/day	6.8	6.4	4.5	4.3
Calcium, %	10.8	11.7	15–17	17.5
Phosphorus, %	6.3	6.5	4.0	7.0
Salt, %	25.3	22.9	22.0	18.5
Magnesium, %	0.86	0.43	5.5	2.7
Potassium, %	0.96	0.88	-	0.1
Copper, ppm	899	767	650	1200
Zinc, ppm	3961	2958	2185	4200

Adapted from Beck and Reuter (2022)[7] with permission.

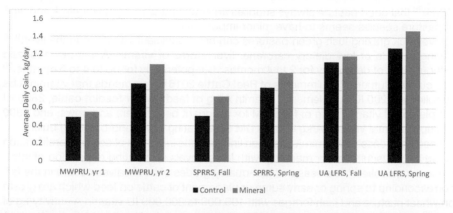

Fig. 1. Response of steers grazing wheat pature to supplemental free-choice mineral supplements compared with controls fed no mineral supplement (MWPRU, [Fieser et al,[33] 2007] and SPPRS Fall and SPRRS Spring [Gunter and Combs,[34] 2019]), or white salt only.(UALFRS [Beck et al,[35] 2021]). (*Adapted from* Beck and Reuter, (2022)[7] with permission.)

Finally, Beck and colleagues (2021)[35] indicated that ADG was numerically increased by 0.1 kg/d during the fall (UA LFRS, Fall; see **Fig. 1**) and significantly increased by 0.19 kg/d during the spring (UA LFRS, Spring; see **Fig. 1**). Summarizing these 6 experiments in 3 widely separate locations shows that a balanced, complete mineral increased gains of steers grazing wheat pasture by an average of 0.15 kg/d.

Vitamins in Small Grain Forages

Vitamins are essential for normal metabolism in physiological functions related to maintenance, growth, development, and reproduction.[36] The vitamins with defined requirements set by the NASEM (2016)[9] include A, D, E. Vitamin K and most water-soluble B vitamins are synthesized by ruminal microflora, so no requirements have been set for cattle in normal production environments.[9] Possible exceptions include vitamin B12 with its deficiency tied directly to cobalt deficiency and concerns regarding polioencephalomalacia in situations with high dietary or water sulfur content[9] resulting in thiamine inefficiency. The following discussion will focus on the fat-soluble vitamins A, D, and E and their supply from fresh growing forages.

Vitamin A

Vitamin A is required for cell differentiation so is important in bone growth, vision, reproduction and growth and differentiation of epithelial tissues.[36] Vitamin A does not occur in plant products but its precursors can be found in several forms including β-carotene, β-cryptoxanthin, and α-carotene. These pro-vitamin A carotenoids are considered to be variable in Vitamin A activity; with 1 mg of β-carotene equal to 400 IU of vitamin A, 1 mg of β-cryptoxanthin being equal to 200 IU of vitamin A, and 1 mg of α-carotene being equal to 200 IU of vitamin A.[37] These precursors occur as orange-yellow pigments in green leaves and all green parts of growing plants are rich in carotene and thus have high vitamin A value, and thus the degree of greenness is a good index of carotene content.[36] The NRC (1984)[38] indicated that fresh wheat forage contained 208,000 carotene vitamin A activity IU/kg of DM. Estimates by Pickworth and colleagues (2012)[37] for fresh tall fescue forage ranged from 34,952 to 45,220 IU vitamin A activity/kg of DM, lending support to the statement from Roche

(1994)[36] that good pasture always supplies an abundant amount of vitamin A and type of pasture species seems to have minor importance.

Livestock grazing lush green pastures can store sufficient vitamin A in the liver.[9,36] During periods of low dietary carotene, liver stores of vitamin A will be mobilized without signs of deficiency for 2 to 4 months[9] but potentially for up to 4 to 6 months.[36] The current Nutrient Requirements of Beef Cattle 2016 recommends that vitamin A be supplied at 2200 IU supplemental vitamin A/kg of feed DM for feedlot cattle, 2800 IU supplemental vitamin A/kg of feed DM for pregnant beef heifers and cows, and 3900 IU supplemental vitamin A/kg of feed DM for lactating cows and breeding bulls.[9]

Feeding excessive vitamin A has been linked to the inhibition of adipose proliferation in the intramuscular fat (or marbling) with lower levels stimulating deposition of intramuscular adipose.[39] The seasonal low-quality grades of beef calves occurs in the fall, corresponding to spring or early summer placement of cattle on feed which are grown on wheat pasture and lush forages with 100,000 to 300,000 IU vitamin A activity/kg of DM.[39] Kohlmeier and Burroughs (1970)40 showed that plasma and liver vitamin A levels of cattle previously grazing wheat pasture entering the feedlot were 1.47 and 3.7-times higher respectively, than plasma and liver levels in cattle previously fed dry forages. The daily depletion rate for vitamin A in plasma was 0.15 μg/dL, taking 140 days for plasma vitamin A to equilibrate between wheat forage and dry hay diets.[40]

Vitamin D

The major function of vitamin D is Ca homeostasis,9 but deficiencies have been linked to immune disfunction43 along with the more commonly known metabolic disease rickets.[41] Vitamin D supplied through the diet or by the irradiation of the body via sunlight,[42] so, in normal conditions it is thought there is little to no need for vitamin D supplementation of cattle in extensive grazing environments, but recent data indicate that necessary rays are emitted year round below the 35° latitude.[42] Jäpelt and Jakobsen (2013)[42] reported vitamin D2 content of perennial ryegrass to be 2 μg/kg of fresh weight. In an assessment of vitamin D concentrations of cows in Florida, Idaho, and Minnesota, all cows were found to have serum 25-hydroxyvitamin D levels above 30 ng/mL, the level thought to indicate adequacy for immune function.[43] Concentrations of 25-hydroxyvitamin D rose from 54 to 58 ng/mL in the spring for cows in northern regions to over 75 ng/mL in the summer.[43] Calves in all locations had average serum concentrations below 20 ng/mL at birth, with concentrations rising to near 50 ng/mL at the end of the summer.[43] Lack of storage depots for vitamin D in land mammalian species indicates there is a potential benefit to supplemental vitamin D over the winter months, more research is needed in this arena. The NASEM (2016)[9] recommended requirement for vitamin D is 275 IU/kg of dietary DM for beef cattle.

Vitamin E

Vitamin E activity is derived from tocopherols and tocotrienols, which are compounds of plant origin.[36] The compound α-tocopherol is the most biologically active and the most predominant vitamin E active compound in feeds and forages.[36] Vitamin E functions as primarily as an intercellular and intracellular antioxidant within cell membranes. Requirements have not been clearly established for beef cattle, as some functions of vitamin E can be fulfilled in part by Se or other antioxidants, but current NASEM (2016)9 guidelines call for 25 to 35 IU/kg dietary DM for finishing cattle and 400 to 500 IU/day for high stressed receiving calves. Selenium is essential in its protection of cell membranes from oxidative erosion as an antioxidant along with vitamin

E, because of its role in the enzyme glutathione peroxidase. Glutathione peroxidase protects membranes from peroxides before they can cause damage, while vitamin E is a fat-soluble antioxidant within the membrane. Vitamin E has a well-known sparing effect on Se,[23,36] which may mask some of the immunological effects of a marginal Se deficiency. Vitamin E is widely distributed in natural feeds with green forages having high levels of α-tocopherol with leaves having 20 to 30 times more α-tocopherol than stems.[36]

Diagnostic Evaluation of Vitamin and Mineral Status

Although fat-soluble vitamins should not be deficient in cattle grazing small grain forages, key understanding of sampling and testing is important. Good diagnostic information on fat-soluble vitamins can be obtained from analysis of either serum or liver samples, but appropriate sample handling is necessary for accurate results. Serum should be separated from the clot as soon as possible and protected from heat and light, which can degrade fat-soluble vitamins. It is critical that liver samples are very fresh, as tissue autolysis can cause the degradation of these vitamins. If the freshness of the sample is in question, a separate sample of formalin-fixed tissue can be submitted for histopathology to ensure that there is no tissue autolysis. If liver tissue autolysis or necrosis is observed, one must assume that at least some of the fat-soluble vitamins have been degraded and any analytical results are artificially low. Thus, deficient liver vitamin content, in the presence of autolysis/necrosis, will not be an accurate reflection of true clinical status. Both serum and liver samples should be maintained frozen for shipment to the testing laboratory.

Mineral deficiencies in cattle were a common finding at the Utah Veterinary Diagnostic Laboratory during the period of 1996 to 2021. The most commonly diagnosed mineral deficiencies in cattle were for copper and selenium, with lesser deficiencies identified for zinc. Some groups of tested cattle had over 80% with deficiencies, as was found for groups of stocker calves tested coming through auction markets in southern Kentucky and southern Missouri. These groups of calves were being tested due to history of poor vaccine efficacy/response and high incidence of infectious diseases.

The best possible means of evaluating mineral status is via testing for specific deficits in mineral-specific proteins or enzymes, but this is generally impractical due to costs, lack of mineral-specific biomarkers, sample handling requirements, or laboratory capabilities.[44] Most minerals have sample specificity where one sample type is generally better than others for evaluation. Serum is generally the best sample type for primary cation and anion macro-minerals, as high body turnover and intracellular to extracellular gradients typically result in relatively consistent tissue concentrations, even with clinical deficiencies. Hepatic tissue is a primary storage tissue for most of the trace minerals. But the status of some trace minerals can be effectively evaluated in both serum and liver.

Although serum or liver mineral analysis are both frequently used for the evaluation of cattle trace mineral status, liver is often the better sample for accurate interpretation of status (**Table 4**). For some minerals that are at much higher content inside red blood cells than in clean serum, hemolysis can artificially increase the serum content and mask a truly deficient content. This is especially true for iron, magnesium, potassium, and zinc, but hemolysis can cause lesser increases for selenium and manganese. Thus, non-hemolyzed samples are critical for certain minerals for accurate and interpretable results. Serum copper is especially problematic for interpretation, as serum content generally does not drop below a normal range until tissue concentrations are severely deficient, and with excessive tissue copper content it does not increase

Table 4
Sample type suitability for the best evaluation of mineral status

	Liver	Serum	Whole Blood	Effects of Sample Hemolysis on Serum Content[a]
Ca	Poor	Best	Poor	Hemolysis can slightly decrease content
Co	Best	Poor[b]	Data Lacking	No Effect
Cu	Best	Poor	Poor	No Effect
Fe	Best	OK if no hemolysis	Data Lacking	Hemolysis can significantly increase content
K	Poor	Best	Poor	Hemolysis can significantly increase content
Mg	Poor	Best	Poor	Hemolysis can slightly increase content
Mn	Best	OK	OK	Hemolysis can slightly increase content
Mo	Best	OK	Data Lacking	No Effect
Na	Poor	Best	Poor	Hemolysis can slightly decrease content
P	Poor	Best	Poor	Hemolysis can increase content
Se	Best	OK if no hemolysis	OK	Hemolysis can slightly increase content
Zn	Best	OK if no hemolysis	Data Lacking	Hemolysis can significantly increase content

[a] The degree is dependent on the severity of the hemolysis.
[b] Low end of serum normal range below testing range for many laboratories.

until it is dumped from liver stores during an acute toxic release. For example, 10 paired serum and liver biopsy samples from the same animals were submitted for testing. All 10 were copper deficient for liver content, but only 1 had a deficient serum content. In another example, 12 cows had potentially toxic liver copper content, but

Table 5
Utah Veterinary Diagnostic Laboratory normal and deficient trace and macro-minerals in cattle - 2021

	Normal Serum Concentration (ppm)	Normal Whole Blood Concentration (ppm)	Normal Wet Weight Liver Concentration (ppm)	Deficient Wet Weight Liver Concentration (ppm)
Ca	80–120	60–90	30–200	NA
Co	< 0.001–0.100	0.001–0.150	0.02–0.200	< 0.01
Cu	0.60–1.5	0.60–1.5	25–100	< 20
Fe	1.0–2.5	300–450	45–300	< 35
K	160–240	800–1200	1400–4000	NA
Mg	18–30	20–70	100–250	NA
Mn	0.002–0.070	0.015–0.090	2.0–6.0	< 1.0
Mo	0.01–0.5	0.01–0.5	0.10–1.40	<0.05
Na	2850–3550	2300–2900	600–3500	NA
P (total)	70–250	200–400	2000–4500	NA
Se	0.08–0.30	0.20–1.20	0.25–0.50	< 0.20
Zn	0.8–2.0	2.0–5.0	25–100	< 20

Partially extracted from Puls (1994).[47]
NA - Liver tissue not applicable to determine systemic status.

were experiencing no clinical abnormalities and all of the serum samples were at the very low end of the normal range.

Often serum is utilized as an easy sample to collect from live animals, but with current analytical technology small liver biopsy samples can also be utilized.[45] A 14-gauge Tru-Cut biopsy needle sample provides between 15 and 20 mg of liver tissue. It is recommended that 2 biopsy samples from each animal be taken for analysis. Samples should be placed into small tubes and frozen. Microcentrifuge tubes work well, as samples can be pushed to the bottom of the tube, limiting air-sample interface and sample drying in transit. The samples should be individually analyzed and not pooled, as animal to animal variability can be important in herd evaluation.

For some trace minerals, normal and deficient ranges are varied, depending on the source of the information.[46] The normal ranges used by the Utah Veterinary Diagnostic Laboratory were partially extracted from published data and partially modified after the evaluation of diagnostic case data with responses to dietary changes (**Table 5**). This data categorizes animals as being deficient in copper, selenium, and zinc at higher liver concentrations than some literature indicates.[46] For these minerals, herds with animal that had mineral concentrations below that listed as deficient responded positively, in terms of incidence of disease, reproductive performance, and growth, when supplemented to be greater than the listed deficiency thresholds in the table.

SUMMARY

Small grain forages provide grazing resources for cattle producers in areas of the United States where cool season perennial grass species do not persist. These lush forages offer the advantages of high protein and digestibility, but both macro and micro mineral needs must be addressed. While the theme of this article is trace minerals, calcium and magnesium deficiencies should be recognized and addressed, especially in lactating cows. Trace mineral content of forages vary considerably, depending on management, group conditions, and soil mineral content. For this reason, small grain forages should be analyzed to accurately formulate mineral supplements. The trace mineral status of cattle grazing small grain forages can be determined by serum analysis, liver biopsy, or submission of liver and kidney samples collected at necropsy. It is extremely important to collect the most appropriate sample for the trace mineral of interest to avoid erroneous interpretation of results.

Small grain forages are rich in vitamins A and E, and vitamin D is supplied through the irradiation of the body via sunlight, therefore supplements with these vitamins is not necessary.

CLINICS CARE POINTS

- In general, small grain pastures can be considered to be very low in Ca, marginal in P, with sufficient Mg. Mg status can be complicated because the high K content of wheat forage interferes with Mg absorption in the gastro-intestinal tract.

- There is considerable variation in the trace mineral composition of small grain forages, depending on management, growth conditions and soil mineral content. There are often deficiencies observed in Cu, Zn and Se.

- Offering a complete mineral increased gains of steers grazing wheat pasture by an average of 0.15 kg/day.

- The vitamins with defined requirements include A, D, E. Vitamin K and most water soluble B vitamins are synthesized by ruminal microflora, so no requirements have been set for cattle in normal production environments. Livestock grazing lush green pastures can store sufficient vitamin A in the liver and during periods of low dietary carotene, liver stores of vitamin A will be mobilized without signs of deficiency for 2 to 4 months. Lack of storage depots for vitamin D in land mammalian species indicates there is potential benefit to supplemental vitamin D over the winter months. Vitamin E is widely distributed in natural feeds with green forages having high levels of α-tocopherol in leaves. In lush growing wheat pasture there is little need for vitamin supplementation.

- Although serum or liver mineral analysis are both frequently used for the evaluation of cattle trace mineral status, liver is often the better sample for accurate interpretation of status. Often serum is utilized as an easy sample to collect from live animals, but with current analytical technology small liver biopsy samples can provide more accurate indcations of status. It is extremely important to collect the most appropriate sample for the trace mineral of interest to avoid erroneous interpretation of true status.

DISCLOSURE

The authors have no conflicts of interest to disclose.

REFERENCES

1. Edwards J, Horn G. First hollow stem: a critical wheat growth state for dual-purpose producers. Crop Soils Mag 2016;49(1):10–4.
2. Fieser BG, Horn GW, Edwards JT, et al. Timing of grazing termination in dual-purpose winter wheat enterprises. Prof Anim Sci 2006;22(3):210–6.
3. Beck PA, Stewart CB, Phillips JM, et al. Effect of species of cool-season annual grass interseeded into bermudagrass sod on the performance of growing calves. J Anim Sci 2007;85:536–44.
4. Beck PA, Hubbell D, Hess T, et al. Case Study: Stocking rate and supplementation of stocker cattle grazing wheat pasture interseeded into bermudagrass in Northern Arkansas. Prof Anim Sci 2008;24:95–9.
5. Beck PA, Stewart CB, Phillips JM, et al. Case Study: Effects of interseeding date of cool-season annual grasses and pre-plant glyphosate application onto a warm-season grass sod on forage production, forage quality, performance of stocker cattle, and net-return. Prof Anim Sci 2011;27:375–84.
6. Beck P, Anders M, Watkins B, et al. Improving the production, environmental, and economic efficiency of the stocker cattle industry in the Southeastern United States. J Anim Sci 2013;91:2456–66.
7. Beck PA, Reuter RR. Nutritional management of calves grazing wheat and small grain pasture. Bovine Pract 2022;56:29–39.
8. Dairy One. Dairy One Feed Composition Library. 2023. Available at: https://dairyone.com/services/forage-laboratory-services/feed-composition-library/Accessed January 18, 2023.
9. NASEM. National Academies of Sciences. Engineering, and Medicine. Nutrient requirements of beef cattle. 8th revised edition. Washington DC: The National Academies Press; 2016.
10. Stewart BA, Grunes DL, Mathers AC, et al. Chemical composition of winter wheat forage grown where grass tetany and bloat occur. Agron J 1981;73:337–47.
11. Kemp A, Hart ML. Grass tetany in grazing milking cows. Netherlands J Anim Sci (NJAS) 1957;5:4–17.
12. Fontenot JP, Allen VG, Bunce GE, et al. Factors influencing magnesium absorption and metabolism in ruminants. J Anim Sci 1989;67:3445–55.

13. Mayland HF, Grunes DL, Lazar VA. Grass tetany hazard of cereal forages based on chemical composition. Agron J 1976;68:665–7.
14. Brown TF, Moser EB, Zeringue ZK. Mineral profile of feedstuffs produced in Louisiana. New Orleans, LA: Southeast Res Sta Ann Rep. Louisiana Agric Exp Sta; 1988. p. 143–7.
15. McCormick ME, Morgan EB, Brown TF, et al. In: Fontenot J, editor. Relationships between silage digestibility and milk production among Holstein cows. Blacksburg, VA: Proc amer forage grassl council; 1990.
16. Brady NC. The nature and properties of soils. 8th edition. New York, NY: Macmillan Publ Co, Inc; 1974.
17. Gunter SA, Finely JW, Stewart CB, et al. Selenium, zinc, and copper status in growing cattle grazing winter pasture on the coastal plain. J Anim Sci 2006; 84(Suppl. 2):37 (Abstr).
18. Puls R. Mineral Levels in Animal Health: Diagnostic Data. In: Clearbrook, British columbia, Canada sherpa int., clearbrook. 1st edition. British Columbia, Canada: Sherpa Int; 1989.
19. Netherlands Committee on Mineral Nutrition. Trace mineral disorders in Dairy cattle. Wageningen, The Netherlands: Center for Agric Publ; 1973.
20. Underwood EJ, Suttle NF. The mineral nutrition of livestock. 3rd edition. New York: CAB International Pub; 1999.
21. Tessman RK, Lakritz J, Tyler JW, et al. Sensitivity and specificity of serum copper determination for detection of copper deficiency in feeder calves. J Am Vet Med Assoc 2001;218:756–60.
22. Beck PA, Gunter SA, Malcolm-Callis KJ, et al. Performance of steers supplemented with copper before and during receiving at the feedlot. Can J Anim Sci 2002;82:87–93.
23. McDowell LR. Minerals for grazing ruminants in tropical regions. 3rd edition. Gainesville, FL: Anim Sci Dept, Univ Florida Bull; 1997.
24. Alloways BJ. Copper and molybdenum in swayback pastures. J Agric Sci 1973; 80:521–4.
25. Ward JD, Spears JW, Kegley EB. Effect of copper level and source (copper lysine vs copper sulfate) on copper status, performance, and immune response in growing steers fed diets with or without supplemental molybdenum and sulfur. J Anim Sci 1993;71:2748–55.
26. Gengelbach GP, Ward JD, Spears JW. Effect of dietary copper, iron, and molybdenum on growth and copper status of beef cows and calves. J Anim Sci 1994; 72:2722–7.
27. Kegley EB, Spears JW. Bioavailability of feed grade copper sources (oxide, sulfate, or lysine) in growing cattle. J Anim Sci 1994;71:2728–34.
28. Miltimore JE, Mason JL. Copper to molybdenum ratio and molybdenum and copper concentrations in ruminant feeds. Can J Anim Sci 1971;51:193–8.
29. Hoelscher JE, Laurent GD. Soil survey of hempstead county, Arkansas. USDA, SCS. Fayetteville, AR: Arkansas Agric Exp Sta; 1979.
30. Russell FC, Duncan DL. Minerals in pasture: Deficiencies and excesses in relation to animal health. Tech Comm Commonwealth Agric Bureaux, No. 15. 1956. Slough: Commonwealth Agric Bureaux.
31. Gunter SA, Beck PA, Phillips JM. Effects of supplementary selenium source on the performance of and blood parameters in beef cows and their calves. J Anim Sci 2003;81:856–64.
32. Beck PA, Wistuba TJ, Davis ME, et al. Case Study: Impact of feeding supplemental organic or inorganic selenium sources to cow-calf pairs on selenium

status and immune responses of weaned beef calves. Prof Anim Sci 2005;21: 114–20.

33. Fieser BG, Horn GW, Edwards JT. Effects of energy, mineral supplementation, or both in combination with monensin on performance of steers grazing winter wheat pasture. J Anim Sci 2007;85(12):3470–80.

34. Gunter SA, Combs FF. Efficacy of mineral supplementation to growing cattle grazing winter wheat pasture in northwestern Oklahoma. Transl Anim Sci 2019; 3(4):1119–32.

35. Beck PA, Foote AP, Galyen WL, et al. Effects of bambermycin or monensin offered in self-fed mineral supplements on performance of growing steer calves grazing small-grain pastures. Appl Anim Sci 2021;37(6):670–80.

36. Vitamin Roche. Nutrition for ruminants. Nutley, NJ. USA: Hoffman-LaRoche Inc.; 1994.

37. Pickworth CL, Loerch SC, Kopec RE, et al. Concentration of pro-vitamin A carotenoids in common beef cattle feedstuffs. J Anim Sci 2012;90:1553–61.

38. National Research Council. Nutrient requirements of beef cattle. 6th edition. Washington DC: National Academy Press; 1984.

39. Pyatt NA, Berger LL. Review: Potential effects of vitamins A and D on marbling deposition in beef cattle. Prof Anim Sci 2005;21:174–81.

40. Kohlmeier RH, Borroughs W. Estimation of critical plasma and liver vitamin A levels in feedlot catle with observations upon influences of body stores and daily dietary requirements. J Anim Sci 1970;30:1012–8.

41. Littledike ET, Goff J. Interactions of calcium, phosphorus, magnesium and vitamin D that influence their status in domestic meat animals. J Anim Sci 1987;65: 1727–43.

42. Jäpelt RB, Jakobsen J. Vitamin D in plants: a review of occurrence, analysis, and biosynthesis. Frontiers Plant Sci 2013;4:1–20.

43. Nelson DC, Powell JL, Price DM, et al. Assessment of serum 25-hydroxyvitamin D concentrations of beef cows and calves across seasons and geographical locations. J Anim Sci 2016;94:3958–65.

44. Hall JO. Appropriate Methods of Diagnosing Mineral Deficiencies in Cattle. Proc the Tri-State Dairy Nutrition Conf; Ft. Wayne, IN; 2006. p. 43–50.

45. Rogers GM, Capucille DJ, Poore MH, et al. Growth performance of cattle following percutaneous liver biopsy utilizing a Schackelford-Courtney biopsy instrument. Bov Pract 2001;35(2):177–84.

46. Spears JW, Brandao VLN, Heldt J. Invited Review: Assessing trace mineral status in ruminants, and factors that affect measurements of trace mineral status. Appl Anim Sci 2022;38(3):252–67.

47. Puls R. Mineral Levels in Animal Health: Diagnostic Data, Second Edition. Sherpa Int: 1994; Clearbrook, British Columbia, Canada Sherpa Int., Clearbrook, British Columbia, Canada.

Vitamins and Trace Minerals in Ruminants
Confinement Feedlot

John J. Wagner, PhD, PAS, Lily N. Edwards-Callaway, PhD,
Terry E. Engle, PhD, PAS*

KEYWORDS

• Feedlot • Performance • Health • Concentrations • Review

KEY POINTS

• Trace minerals and vitamins are key components in feedlot diets.
• Many factors can impact trace mineral and vitamin absorption and metabolism.
• Supplementing trace minerals and vitamins above requirements may not improve feedlot cattle performance, health, or carcass characteristics.

INTRODUCTION

Trace minerals and vitamins are essential dietary components for domestic livestock species. They are integral components for normal carbohydrate, lipid, and protein metabolism and have been shown to be involved in hormone production, immunity, oxidation/reduction reactions, and cellular homeostasis. However, the functions of trace minerals and vitamins in metabolic processes are extremely complex.

In general, trace minerals function primarily as activators or components of enzyme systems within cells by assisting with enzyme structural integrity and/or substrate binding. Enzymes involved in protection of cells from oxidative stress, electron transport, oxygen transport, bone metabolism, gene expression, and nutrient metabolism all have been shown to require certain trace elements for proper function. The trace minerals typically supplemented to feedlot cattle diets are cobalt (Co), copper (Cu), iodine (I), manganese (Mn), selenium (Se), and zinc (Zn). Although chromium (Cr) is not considered an essential nutrient in the National Academies of Sciences, Engineering, and Medicine (NASEM),[1] it is being included in some feedlot diet.

Vitamins are classified as either water- or lipid-soluble and have been shown to function in cellular differentiation, immunity, maintenance of redox status, bone

Department of Animal Science, Colorado State University, 350 West Pitkin Street, Fort Collins, CO 80523, USA
* Corresponding author.
E-mail address: terry.engle@colostate.edu

Vet Clin Food Anim 39 (2023) 505–516
https://doi.org/10.1016/j.cvfa.2023.06.005
vetfood.theclinics.com

remodeling, vision, blood clotting, neural tissue development, and energy metabolism. Water-soluble vitamins are usually synthesized in appropriate amounts by rumen microorganisms (eg, B vitamins) or endogenously (eg, vitamin C) to meet the animal's needs and thus are rarely supplemented in feedlot diets. Vitamins D and K are lipid-soluble vitamins that are synthesized by UV light interaction with the skin or by microorganisms in the rumen, respectively, and are not typically supplemented in feedlot cattle diets in the United States. However, the lipid-soluble vitamin A and to a lesser extent vitamin E (depending on the basal dietary ingredient concentrations of vitamin E) are supplemented in feedlot diets.

There are many factors that could impact an animal's response to trace mineral and vitamin supplementation, such as the dose and duration of supplementation, physiologic status of an animal, the absence or presence of dietary antagonists, basal diet trace mineral and vitamin concentrations, environmental factors, rumen health, and the degree of stress. Therefore, the intent of this review is to discuss (1) the functions and requirements of trace minerals and vitamins that are commonly supplemented to feedlot cattle; (2) the impact of mineral dose on growth performance and carcass characteristics; (3) the factors that may impact mineral and vitamin metabolism and/or dietary requirements; and (4) the current trace mineral and vitamin supplementation concentrations used by consulting nutritionists in the United States for feedlot cattle.

Topics such as evaluating the impact of environment, trace mineral source, gestation, lactation, and species (goats and sheep) are covered in other articles in this issue of *Veterinary Clinics of North America: Food Animal Practice* on Vitamins and Trace Minerals in Ruminants.

TRACE MINERALS
Cobalt

Currently, there is no known metabolic requirement specifically for Co in beef cattle. However, because Co is required by ruminal microorganism to produce vitamin B12, Co is considered a dietary essential element for ruminants. In a normal, healthy functioning rumen, microorganisms are capable of supplying enough vitamin B12 to meet the animal's vitamin B12 requirements.[2] There are 2 known vitamin B12–dependent enzymes that occur in beef cattle: methylmalonyl CoA mutase and 5-methyltetrahydrofolate homocysteine methyltransferase (methionine synthase).[2] These vitamin B12–dependent enzymes are involved in (1) propionate incorporation into intermediates involved in gluconeogenesis and (2) methyl group transfer and methionine homeostasis, respectively.[2]

The current dietary requirement for Co is 0.15 mg Co/kg dry matter (DM) with a maximum tolerable concentration of 25 mg Co/kg DM.[1] The wide range between the requirement and maximum tolerable concentrations indicates that cattle can tolerate greater than 100 times their dietary requirement. In situations of low dry matter intake (eg, light weight, stressed, receiving cattle) and/or cattle experiencing digestive upsets (eg, acidosis), the conversion of Co to vitamin B12 in the rumen may be compromised, and additional Co and/or vitamin B12 supplementation may be warranted.[1] In the most recent survey of US consulting feedlot nutritionists (representing more than 14 million feedlot cattle on feed), the mode for Co inclusion into receiving and finishing diet was 0.20 mg Co/kg DM.[3]

However, the range for Co inclusion for receiving and finishing diets was 0.0 to 5.0 and 0.0 to 3.0 mg Co/kg DM, respectively. The reason for the inclusion of excessively high concentrations of Co by some consulting nutritionists was not discussed by Samuelson and colleagues.[3]

Feedlot growth responses to varying doses of dietary Co have been variable. Using intact male Simmental cattle fed a corn silage—based diet supplemented with a protein-energy concentrate, maximal plasma and liver B12 concentrations, average daily gains, and dry matter intakes were observed in diets containing 0.26, 0.24, 0.12, and 0.17 mg Co/kg DM, respectively.[4,5] Tiffany and colleagues[6] supplemented 0.0, 0.05, 0.10, and 1.0 mg Co/kg DM to growing and finishing steers (basal diets contained 0.04 mg Co/kg DM) and reported that Co supplementation had no impact on growth performance during the growing phase of the experiment. However, steers receiving supplemental Co had greater DM intake, average daily gains, plasma glucose, final body weights, and hot carcass weights compared with the controls. Similarly, in a dose response experiment, Sharman and colleagues[7] reported that finishing steers supplemented with 1.0 mg Co/kg DM (basal finishing diet contained 0.05 mg Co/kg DM) tended to have greater average daily gains and had greater carcass yield grades, back fat thickness, and serum, liver, and longissimus muscle concentrations than steers receiving 0.10 mg Co/kg DM. In contrast, Tiffany and Spears[8] reported no differences in plasma and liver vitamin B12 concentrations or overall average daily gains and dry matter intakes when supplemental Co was increased from 0.05 to 0.15 mg Co/kg DM. Limited research also suggests that ruminants receiving barley-based diets may have a higher dietary Co requirement than animals receiving corn-based diets. This may be due to a reduction in microbial methylmalonyl-CoA mutase activity in barley-fed ruminants.[8–10] Collectively, based on in vitro and in vivo experiments, the Co requirement for finishing cattle receiving corn-based diets is 0.15 mg Co/kg DM but could be higher for cattle fed a barley-based diet.[4–6,11,12]

Copper

Cu is a dietary essential element required by beef cattle and functions as an integral component in numerous enzymes involved in energy, protein, and lipid metabolism. Cellular respiration, cross-linking of connective tissue, central nervous system formation, and immune function have been shown to be altered during a Cu deficiency.[13,14]

The dietary requirement for growing and finishing cattle is 10 mg Cu/kg DM with a maximum tolerable concentration of 40 mg Cu/kg DM.[1] Cattle are known to be more susceptible to Cu toxicosis that nonruminants. Binding proteins in the liver prevent free Cu from inducing cellular damage, but the liver has a low capacity to incorporate Cu into bile for excretion when compared with nonruminants. Therefore, feeding elevated Cu concentration to beef cattle can cause an accumulation in liver Cu concentrations, which could lead to hemolytic crisis if binding capacity is exceeded.[15,16]

Based on the consulting nutritionist survey conducted by Samuelson and colleagues,[3] the mode for Cu supplementation in receiving and finishing diets was 20 mg Cu/kg DM with a range of 20 to 60 mg Cu/kg DM and 10.0 to 40.0 mg Cu/kg DM for receiving and finishing diets, respectively. However, controlled experiments examining the impact of Cu dose on growth performance and carcass characteristics have reported positive, negative, and no effect of Cu supplementation at doses ranging from 0 to 20 mg of supplemental Cu/kg DM.[17–22]

The reason for the variability in growth performance and carcass merit responses to dietary Cu supplementation may be due to dietary Cu antagonists. Numerous antagonists in the diet and/or water can reduce the availability of dietary Cu, such as elevated concentrations of Fe, Mo, S, and Zn.[23–31] Pogge and colleagues conducted a meta-analysis to evaluate the impact of Cu, molybdenum (Mo), and sulfur (S) from 12 published feedlot experiments. The investigators reported that dietary Cu concentrations impacted Cu status but had no impact on growing and finishing cattle performance. However, as the ratio of Cu:Mo increased (more dietary Cu and less Mo), mineral status and average daily gain increased. Although there are no definitive data in the literature identifying the appropriate minimum Cu:Mo ratio, a Cu:Mo ratio greater than or equal to 3:1 is recommended.[14] Furthermore, as the dietary concentration of S increased, mineral status, average daily gain, and feed efficiency decreased.[30] These data indicate that it is important to understand Cu antagonists in the diet in order to meet the animal's requirement and that supplementing concentrations greater than 10 mg Cu/kg DM may be warranted in certain situations when dietary Mo and S concentrations exceed requirements.

Chromium

Cr was first shown to be essential for mammals by modulating the impact of insulin on certain tissues.[1,32] Following the initial discovery, Cr has been reported to influence carbohydrate, protein, and lipid metabolism,[33–37] immunity (Burton and colleagues, 1993), and possibly attenuate heat stress in dairy cows.[38]

In 2019, Budde and colleagues[39] supplemented feedlot steers with 0.25 mg Cr/kg DM and 90 mg Zn/kg DM and reported improved final body weights, average daily gains, and hot carcass weights when compared with steers receiving no supplemental Cr and 90 mg of supplemental Zn/kg DM. Earlier work by Bernhard and colleagues[40] reported a linear increase in live animal performance in newly received feedlot cattle when Cr was supplemented at 0.0, 0.1, 0.2, and 0.3 mg Cr/kg DM.[41] Kneeskern and colleagues reported that supplemented feedlot steers with extremely high concentrations of Cr (13.47 mg Cr/kg DM) increased yield grade, tended to increase longissimus muscle area, and tended to decrease marbling score and intramuscular fat deposition. The exact mechanism whereby Cr may be increasing growth in beef cattle is not fully understood. The addition of 0.4 mg Cr/kg DM to stressed feedlot cattle increased glucose clearance rate following intravenous glucose administration[42] and increased insulin sensitivity.[43,44] Increasing glucose metabolism by tissues may result in improved tissue growth.

The impact of Cr supplementation to feedlot cattle on immune function has been variable. Supplementing stressed beef cattle with 0.4 mg Cr/kg DM had no impact on immune response to a foreign antigen.[45,46] However, supplementing newly weaned calves with 0.5 mg Cr/kg DM for 30 days postarrival to the feedlot increased antibody titers to certain vaccine components but on to others.[47]

The reason for the variable responses of Cr supplementation on immune responses in beef cattle is unclear. Factors that contribute to the inconsistent findings between studies may include the following: (1) the initial Cr status of the animals; (2) the amount of available Cr in the control diet; (3) the form of Cr supplemented; (4) analytical errors; and (5) the type or degree of stress imposed on the animal.[48]

Iodine

The thyroid hormones (T3 and T4), which regulate energy metabolism, require I to function appropriately.[1] A deficiency in I causes reduced growth rate, impaired reproduction, low birth weights, goiter, and death.[1] The I requirement for beef cattle is not well defined but has been estimated to be approximately 0.50 mg/kg DM.[1,49] Goitrogenic compounds and ambient temperature have been reported to alter I metabolism.[14] The maximum tolerable concentration for I is 50 mg I/kg DM.[15,16] The mode for I inclusion into receiving and finishing diet by consulting feedlot nutritionists[3] was 1.0 and 0.50 mg I/kg DM for receiving and finishing diets, respectively.

Ethylenediamine dihydroiodide (EDDI), a common I source, has been used to prevent foot rot in beef cattle. However, the dose of EDDI needed to prevent foot rot is excessively greater than dietary requirements and has variable impacts on controlling this disease.[1]

Currently, the Food and Drug Administration[50] has set a maximum of less than 50.0 mg of EDDI that can be fed per animal daily.[1]

Manganese

To date, there have been 3 Mn-dependent enzymes (metalloenzymes) identified in mammals: Mn-superoxide dismutase, pyruvate carboxylase, and arginase.[51] These 3 enzymes are responsible for reducing the risk of peroxidation damage in the mitochondria, gluconeogenesis, and urea metabolism, respectively.[14] Mn has also been identified as an essential component for proper bone and cartilage formation and growth.[52] Leach reported that Mn is essential in the activation of glycosyltransferases that are partly responsible for mucopolysaccharide synthesis. Without these structural components of cartilage, skeletal defects can result. Therefore, Mn deficiency can potentially lead to a decrease in overall animal growth.[53]

The Mn requirements for growing and finishing beef cattle are 20 mg Mn/kg DM.[1,54,55] The mode for Mn inclusion in feedlot diets reported by consulting nutritionists in the United States was 50 mg Mn/kg DM for both receiving and finishing diets with ranges of 20 to 140 mg Mn/kg DM for receiving diets and 20 to 100 mg Mn/kg DM for finishing diets.[3] The maximum tolerable concentration for Mn is 1000 mg Mn/kg DM. The reason for supplementing greater Mn concentrations in feedlot diets reported by consulting feedlot nutritionist is unclear. However, high dietary concentrations of calcium (Ca), phosphorus (P), and iron (Fe) have been reported to interfere with Mn availability,[26,56–58] and therefore, diets may need to be supplemented with higher concentrations of Mn under these conditions.

Selenium

Se is needed for appropriate growth and immune function in beef cattle. Briefly, Se is an integral component in numerous selenoproteins that function primarily as antioxidants. Furthermore, 5'deiodinase (types 1–3) is an Se-dependent enzyme that converts the thyroid hormone T4 to the more bioactive thyroid hormone T3.[13,14] Deficiencies in Se can cause peroxidation of skeletal and heart muscle, anemia, impaired immune response, altered T4 and T3 ratios, and reduced growth in cattle.[14,48,59,60]

The dietary Se requirement for feedlot cattle is 0.1 mg Se/kg DM.[1] Although extremely rare in feedlot situations, Se toxicosis can occur regionally when cattle graze Se accumulator plants growing on seleniferous range in the western United States; therefore, the maximum allowable amount of Se that can legally be supplemented in beef cattle diets is 0.3 mg Se/kg DM.[1,61] The mode for supplemental Se in receiving and finishing diets reported in the consulting feedlot nutrition survey was 0.30 mg Se/kg DM.[3] Two beef cattle growing/finishing experiments reported that supplementing Se well above NASEM[1] concentrations does not improve performance or carcass characteristics.[62,63]

Zinc

Zn functions in numerous enzymes as either a structural component or an activator and therefore plays a role in gene expression, growth, reproduction, immunity, vitamin metabolism, and many other processes.[13,14,64–70] The dietary requirement of Zn for growing and finishing feedlot cattle is 30 mg Zn/kg DM.[1] In the most recent survey of consulting feedlot nutritionists, the mode for Zn supplementation to receiving and finishing diets was 100 mg Zn/kg DM with a range of 34 to 175 mg Zn/kg DM across receiving and finishing diets.[3]

The reason for the wide range in supplemental Zn concentrations describe above may be due to the variable growth and carcass characteristics responses to elevated supplemental Zn reported in the literature. Current growth technologies, such as anabolic implants and beta-agonists, increase growth efficiency, in part, by increasing protein accretion in cattle.[71,72] Because Zn is involved in protein synthesis and gene transcription, many researchers have investigated the impact of increasing dietary Zn alone or in combination with growth implants and beta-agonists on growth performance and carcass characteristics in cattle.

Collectively, results from these types of experiments have been extremely variable.[73] Van Bibber-Krueger and colleagues reported no impact of Zn dose on feedlot heifer performance or carcass characteristics when heifers were fed Zn supplemented at 0, 30, 60, or 90 mg of Zn/kg DM (basal diet contained 51.4 mg Zn.kg DM) for 144 days. Similar results were reported by Messersmith and colleagues[74] in heifers supplemented with 30 or 100 mg Zn/kg DM (basal finishing diet contained 68 mg/Zn/kg DM) for 168 days. Zn supplementation at 100, 150, and 180 mg Zn/kg DM (basal diet contained 39 mg Zn/kg DM) to steers administered an anabolic implant at the beginning of the experiment and a beta-agonist at the end of the finishing period increased average daily gain through 70 days on feed and increased carcass yield grade but had no impact on overall feedlot performance or other carcass measurements over the entire 98-day experiment, when compared with the nonsupplemented controls.[75] Similar results were obtained by Wellmann and colleagues[76] when steers were supplemented with either 0 or 200 mg Zn/kg DM (basal diet contained 92.6 mg Zn/kg DM); average daily gain and gain:feed were improved from day 80 to 111 (beta-agonist feeding period) in Zn-supplemented steers, but overall animal performance and carcass characteristics were similar across treatments.

Limited research in ruminants examining the influence of Zn supplementation on immune function and disease resistance has been conducted. Although data are limited and variable, Galyean and colleagues[77] reported that increasing the concentration of supplemental Zn from 30- to 100-mg/kg diet tended to reduce morbidity from respiratory diseases in newly weaned stressed (by transport) calves. Supplementing Zn at 25 mg Zn/kg DM to a basal receiving/growing diet containing 33 mg Zn/kg DM improved average daily gains over the 84-day growing period but had no impact on overall performance at the end of the finishing phase. However, supplemental Zn did improve carcass quality grade. These data indicate that Zn requirements for receiving/growing cattle may be greater to optimize growth and disease resistance than for finishing cattle.[78] However, others have reported no impact on performance or health parameters in stressed cattle supplemented with varying concentrations of Zn.[79,80]

SUPPLEMENTING COMBINATIONS OF TRACE MINERALS ABOVE REQUIREMENTS

Several research groups have compared the impact of supplementing elevated concentrations (above the NASEM[1] requirements) of Co, Cu, Mn, Zn, I, Se, and Zn (concurrently) on feedlot cattle performance and carcass characteristics. Results of these experiments have been highly variable, and caution should be taken when comparing experiments. Increasing trace mineral concentrations above published requirements does not always improve feedlot performance and carcass characteristics[81–83] but has been reported to increase dry matter intake and average daily gain during certain intervals of the feeding period.[84] The variability in animal numbers, dietary ingredients, growth technologies used, basal dietary mineral concentrations, and basal dietary availability of trace minerals[85] make comparing these types of experiments difficult.

VITAMINS

Vitamins have been shown to function in cellular differentiation, immunity, maintenance of redox status, bone remodeling, vision, blood clotting, neural tissue development, and energy metabolism.[13,14] Beef cattle can endogenously synthesize vitamin C via the glucuronic pathway in the liver, and bacteria in the rumen can synthesize vitamin K and water-soluble vitamins in amounts that meet the animal's requirement. Therefore, water-soluble vitamins and vitamin K are not typically supplemented to feedlot cattle diets unless rumen function is compromised by shipping stress or dietary antagonists. If this occurs, water-soluble vitamins and vitamin K may be supplemented. The most common example of this scenario is the supplementation of thiamine when S-containing corn processing coproducts, such as distillers grains, are fed. Interestingly, feeding protected vitamin C to feedlot cattle has been reported to improve marbling in feedlot cattle fed diets containing elevated sulfur.[86]

Because of the low content of β-carotene in in most grains, vitamin A is commonly supplemented to feedlot cattle diets. The vitamin A requirement for feedlot cattle is 2200 IU/kg.[1,87–92] The latest consulting feedlot nutritionist survey reported a mode for vitamin A supplementation of 3000 and 2000 IU/kg DM for receiving and finishing cattle, respectively.[3]

Most feedlot cattle in the United States are fed in open lots exposed to direct sunlight, and therefore, vitamin D is not routinely supplemented. However, vitamin D supplementation for cattle fed in total confinement may be warranted. Vitamin E requirements have not been well established for beef cattle. Depending on the vitamin E concentration in the basal dietary ingredients, vitamin E may or not be supplemented in feedlot diets. The NASEM[1] has estimated the vitamin E requirements to be between 15 and 60 IU/kg DM for cattle and may be higher for newly received, stressed calves. The latest consulting feedlot nutritionist survey reported a mode for supplemental vitamin D of 0.0 for both receiving and finishing diets and a vitamin E mode of 20 IU/kg DM and 0.0 IU/kg DM for receiving and finishing diets, respectively.[3]

CLINICS CARE POINTS

- Analyze feed and water routinely for common trace mineral antagonists.
- When formulating diets for trace minerals and vitamins, try to understand the availability of trace minerals and vitamins from basal feed ingredients.
- When assessing the impact of trace minerals on feedlot cattle growth and carcass characteristics, remember that feeding excessive amounts of certain minerals can impact the absorption and metabolism of other nutrients.

DISCLOSURES

The authors have no conflicts of interest.

ACKNOWLEDGEMENT

Claire Okoren, BS, gave significant contribution to the article.

REFERENCES

1. NASEM. National Academies of Sciences, Engineering, and Medicine). In: Nutrient requirements of beef cattle. 8th Revised edition. Washington, DC: The National Academies Press; 2016.
2. Smith RM. Cobalt. In: Mertz W, editor. Trace elements in human and animal nutrition. New York: Academic Press; 1987. p. 143–83.
3. Samuelson KL, Hubbert ME, Galyean ML, et al. Nutritional recommendations of feedlot consulting nutritionists: The 2015 New Mexico State and Texas Tech University survey. J Anim Sci 2016;94:2648–63.
4. Schwarz FJ, Kirchgessner M, Stangl GI. Cobalt requirement of beef cattle-feed intake and growth at different levels of cobalt supply. J Anim Physiol Anim Nutr 2000;83:121–31.
5. Stangl GI, Schwarz FJ, Müller J, et al. Evaluation of the cobalt requirement of beef cattle based on vitamin B12, folate, homocysteine and methylmalonic acid. Br J Nutr 2000;84:645–53.
6. Tiffany ME. Cobalt requirements in growing and finishing cattle based on performance, vitamin B12 status, and metabolite concentrations. Raleigh: Ph.D. Dissertation. North Carolina State University; 2003.
7. Sharman ED, Wagner JJ, Larson CK, et al. The effects of trace mineral source on performance and health of newly received steers and the impact of cobalt concentration on performance and lipid metabolism during the finishing phase. Prof Anim Sci 2008;24:430–8.
8. Tiffany ME, Spears JW. Differential responses to dietary cobalt in finishing steers fed corn- versus barley-based diets. J Anim Sci 2005;83:2580–9.
9. Kennedy DG, Cannavan A, Molloy A, et al. Methylmalonyl-CoA mutase (EC 5.4.99.2) and methionine synthetase (EC 2.1.1.13) in the tissues of cobalt-vitamin B12 deficient sheep. Br J Nutr 1990;64:721–32.
10. Kennedy DG, Young PB, McCaughey WJ, et al. Rumen succinate production may ameliorate the effects of cobalt-vitamin B-12 deficiency on methylmalonyl CoA mutase in sheep. J Nutr 1991;121:1236–42.
11. Tiffany ME, Fellner V, Spears JW. Influence of cobalt concentration on vitamin B12 production and fermentation of mixed ruminal microorganisms in continuous culture-flow through fermenters. J Anim Sci 2006;84:635–40.
12. Spears JW, Weiss WP. Invited Review: Mineral and vitamin nutrition in ruminants. Prof Anim Sci 2014;30:180–91.
13. McDowell LR. Minerals in animal and human nutrition. San Diego, CA: Academic Press Inc. Harcourt Brace Jovanovich Publishers; 1992. ISBN 0-12-483369-1.
14. Underwood EJ, Suttle NF. In: The mineral nutrition of livestock. 3rd edition. Wallingford, Oxon, UK: CABI Publishing, CAB International; 1999.
15. NRC. Mineral tolerance of domestic animals. Washington, D.C.: National Academy of Sciences; 1980. https://doi.org/10.17226/25.
16. NRC. Mineral tolerance of domestic animals. Washington, D.C: National Academy of Sciences; 2005. https://doi.org/10.17226/11309.
17. Ward JD, Spears JW. Long-term effects of consumption of low-copper diets with or without supplemental molybdenum on copper status, performance , and carcass characteristics of cattle. J Anim Sci 1997;75:3057–65.
18. Engle TE, Spears JW. Dietary copper effects on lipid metabolism, performance, and ruminal fermentation in finishing steers. J Anim Sci 2000a;78:2452–8.

19. Engle TE, Spears JW. Effects of copper concentration and source on performance and copper status of growing and finishing steers. J Anim Sci 2000b; 78:2446–51.

20. Engle TE, Spears JW, Fellner V, et al. Effects of soybean oil and dietary copper on ruminal and tissue lipid metabolism in finishing steers. J Anim Sci 2000a;78:2713–21.

21. Engle TE, Spears JW. Performance, carcass characteristics, and lipid metabolism in growing and finishing Simmental steers fed varying concentrations of copper. J Anim Sci 2001;79:2920–5.

22. Lee SH, Engle TE, Hossner KL. Effects dietary copper on the expression of lipogenic genes and metabolic hormones in steers. J Anim Sci 2002;80:1999–2005.

23. Suttle NF. Effects of organic and inorganic sulfur on the availability of dietary copper to sheep. Br J Nutr 1974;32:559–68.

24. Suttle NF. The interactions between copper, molybdenum and sulfur in ruminant nutrition. Annu Rev Nutr 1991;11:121–40.

25. Smart ME, Cohen R, Christensen DA, et al. The effects of sulfate removal from the drinking water on the plasma and liver copper and zinc concentrations of beef cows and their calves. Can J Anim Sci 1986;66:669–80.

26. Spears JW. Trace mineral bioavailability in ruminants. J Nutr 2003;133:1506S–9S.

27. Hansen SL, Spears JW. Bioaccessibility of iron form soils is increased by silage fermentation. J Dairy Sci 2009;92:2896–905.

28. Felix TL, Weiss WP, Fluharty FL, et al. Effects of copper supplementation on feedlot performance, carcass characteristics, and rumen sulfur metabolism of growing cattle fed diets containing 60% dried distillers grains. J Anim Sci 2012;90:2710–6.

29. Kessler KL, Olsen KC, Wright CL, et al. Effects of supplemental molybdenum on animal performance, liver copper concentrations, ruminal hydrogen sulfide concentrations, and the appearance of sulfur and molybdenum toxicity in steers receiving fiber-based diets. J Anim Sci 2012;90:5005–12.

30. Dias RS, Lopez S, Montanholi TR, et al. A meta-analysis of the effect of dietary copper, molybdenum, and sulfur on plasma and liver copper, weight gain, and feed conversion in growing-finishing cattle. J Anim Sci 2013;91:5714–23.

31. Pogge DJ, Drewnoski ME, Hansen SL. Feeding ferric ammonium citrate to decrease the risk of sulfur toxicity: Effects on trace mineral absorption and status of beef steers. J Anim Sci 2014;92:4005–13.

32. Schwarz K, Mertz W. Chromium (III) and the glucose tolerance factor. Arch Biochem Biophys 1959;85:292–5.

33. Mertz W. Chromium in human nutrition: A review. J Nutr 1993;123:626–33.

34. Abraham AB, Brooks BA, Eylath U. Chromium and cholesterol-induced arteriosclerosis in rabbits. Ann Nutr Metab 1991;35:203–7.

35. Okada S, Suzuki M, Ohba H. Enhancement of ribonucleic acids synthesis by chromium (III) in mouse liver. J Inorg Biochem 1983;19:95–103.

36. Kornegay ET, Wang Z, Wood CM, et al. Supplemental chromium picolinate influences nitrogen balance, dry matter digestibility, and carcass traits in growing and finishing pigs. J Anim Sci 1997;75:1319–23.

37. Burton JL, Mallard BA, Mowat DN. Effects of supplemental chromium on immune responses of periparturient and ealry latation dairy cows. J Anim Sci 1993;71:1532–9.

38. Zhang FJ, Weng XG, Wang JF, et al. Effects of temperature-humidity index and chromium supplementation on antioxidant capacity, heat shock protein 72, and cytokine response of lactation cows. J Anim Sci 2014;92:3026–34.

39. Budde AM, Sellins K, Lloyd KE, et al. Effect of zinc source and concentration and chromium supplementation on performance and carcass characteristics in feedlot steers. J Anim Sci 2019;97:1286–95.

40. Bernhard BC, Burdick NC, Rounds W, et al. Chromium supplementation alters the performance and health of feedlot cattle during the receiving period and enhances their metabolic response to a lipopolysaccharide challenge. J Anim Sci 2012;90:3879–88.

41. Kneeskern SG, Dilger AC, Loerch AC, et al. Effects of chromium supplementation to feedlot steers on growth performance, insulin sensitivity, and carcass characteristics. J Anim Sci 2016;94:217–26.

42. Kegley EB, Spears JW. Immune response, glucose metabolism, and performance of stressed feeder calves fed inorganic or organic chromium. J Anim Sci 1995;73:2721–6.

43. Stahlhut HS, Whisnant CS, Lloyd KE, et al. Effect of chromium supplementation and copper status on glucose and lipid metabolism in Angus and Simental beef cows. Amim Feed Sci Technol 2006;128:253–65.

44. Spears JW, Whisnant SC, Huntington GB, et al. Chromium propionate enhances insulin sensitivity in growing cattle. J Dairy Sci 2012;95:2037–45.

45. Kegley EB, Spears JW, Brown TT. Effects of shipping and chromium supplementation on performance, immune response, and disease resistance of steers. J Anim Sci 1997;75:1956–64.

46. Arthington JD, Corah LR, Minton JE, et al. Supplemental dietary chromium does not influence ACTH, cortisol, or immune responses in young claves inoculated with bovine herpesvirus-1. J Anim Sci 1997;75:217–23.

47. Burton JL, Mallard BA, Mowat DN. Effects of supplemental chromium on antibody responses of newly weaned feedlot calves to immunization with infectious bovine rhinotracheitis and parainfluenza 3 virus. Can J Vet Res 1994;58:148–51.

48. Spears JW. Micronutrients and immune function in cattle. Proc Nutr Soc 2000; 59:1–8.

49. ARC(Agricultural Research Council). The nutrient requirements of ruminant livestock. Slough, U.K.: Commonwealth Agricultural Bureaux; 1980.

50. United States FDA Compliance Policy Guide. 2000. CPG sec. 651.100 ethylenediamine dihydroiodide (EDDI). https://www.fda.gov/regulatory-information/search-fda-guidance-documents/cpg-sec-651100- ethylenediamine-dihydroiodide-eddi. Accessed February 14, 2023.

51. Leach RM, Harris ED. Manganese. In: O'Dell BL, Sunde RA, editors. Handbook of nutritionally essential mineral elements. New York: Marcel Dekker, Inc.; 1997. p. 335–55.

52. Leach RM Jr. Role of manganese in mucopolysaccharide metabolism. Fed Proc 1971;30:991–1004.

53. Prasad AS. Trace Metals in Growth and Sexual Maturation. In: Rennert OM, Chan WY, editors. Developmental aspect. Metabolism of trace metals in man, 1. Florida: CRC Press Inc.; 1984. p. 79–97.

54. Legleiter LR, Spears JW, Lloyd KE. Influence of dietary manganese on performance, lipid metabolism, and carcass composition of growing and finishing steers. J Anim Sci 2005;83:2434–9.

55. Hansen SL, Spears JW, Lloyd KE, et al. Growth, reproductive performance, and manganese status of heifers fed varying concentrations of manganese. J Anim Sci 2006;84:3375–80.

56. Hawkins GE Jr, Wise GH, Matrone G, et al. Manganese in the nutrition of young dairy cattle fed different levels of calcium and phosphorus. J Dairy Sci 1955;38: 536–47.

57. Dyer IA, Cassatt WA, Rao RR. Manganese deficiency in the etiology and deformed calves. Bioscience 1964;14:31–2.

58. Hansen SL, Ashwell MS, Moeser AJ, et al. High dietary iron reduces transporters involved in iron and manganese metabolism and increases intestinal permeability in calves. J Dairy Sci 2010;93:656–65.

59. Arthur JR, Beckett GJ. New metabolic roles for selenium. Proc Nutr Soc 1994;53: 615–24.

60. Stabel JR, Spears JW, Brown TT. Effect of copper deficiency on tissue, blood characteristics, and immune function of calves challenged with infectious bovine rhinotracheitis virus and Pasteurella hemolytica. J Anim Sci 1993;71:1247–55.

61. United States, Department of Health and Human Services, FDA. 2022. Subchapter E, animal drugs, feeds, and related products, selenium, code of federal regulations-21cfr § 573.920. https://www.ecfr.gov/current/title-21/chapter-I/subchapter-E/part-573/subpart-B/section- 573.920. Accessed February 14, 2023.

62. Hintze KJ, Lardy GP, Marchello MJ, et al. Selenium accumulation in beef: Effect of dietary selenium and geographical area of animal origin. J Agric Food Chem 2002;50:3938–42.

63. Lawler TL, Taylor JB, Finlet JW, et al. Effect of supranational and organically bound selenium on performance, carcass characteristics, and selenium distribution in finishing steers. J Anim Sci 2004;82:1488–93.

64. Mills DF, Chesters JK. Problems in the execution of nutritional and metabolic experiments with trace element deficient animals. In: Mills CF, editor. Trace element metabolism in Animals. Edinburgh and London: E.& S. Livingstone; 1969. p. 39–50.

65. Smith KT, Failla ML, Cousins RJ. Identification of albumin as the plasma carrier for zinc absorption by perfused rat intestine. Biochem J 1979;184:627–33.

66. Hambidge KM, Casey CE, Krebs NF. In: Mertz W, editor. Zinc. Page 1 in Trace elements in human and animal nutrition. vol. 2. New York: Academic Press; 1986.

67. Apgar J. Zinc and reproduction: an update. J Nutr Biochem 1992;3:266–77.

68. Chesters JK. In: O'Dell BL, Sunde RA, editors. Zinc. Handbook of nutritionally essential mineral elements. New York, New York: Marcel Dekker Inc.; 1997.

69. George MH, Nockels CG, Stanton TL, et al. Effect of source and amount of zinc, copper, manganese, and cobalt fed to stressed heifers on feedlot performance and immune function. Prof Anim Sci 1997;13:84–9.

70. Galyean ML, Perino LJ, Duff GC. Interaction of cattle health/immunity and nutrition. J Anim Sci 1999;77:1120–34.

71. Duckett SK, Pratt SL. Anabolic implants and meat quality. J Anim Sci 2014; 92:3–9.

72. Lean IJ, Thompson JM, Dunshea FR. A meta-analysis of zilpaterol and ractopamine effects on feedlot performance, carcass traits and shear strength of meat in cattle. PLoS One 2014;9:e115904.

73. Van Bibber-Krueger CL, Cajh CI, Naratanan SK, et al. Effects of supplemental zinc sulfate on growth performance, carcass characteristics, and antimicrobial resistance in feedlot heifers. J Anim Sci 2019;97:424–36.

74. Messersmith EM, Smerchek DT, Hansen SL. The crossroads between zinc and steroidal implanted-inuced growth of beef cattle. Animals 2019;11:1914–34.

75. Messersmith EM, Smerchek DT, Hansen SL. Effects of increasing supplemental zinc in beef feedlot steers administered a steroidal implant and beta agonist. Transl Anim Sci 2022;6:1–10.

76. Wellmann KB, Baggerman JO, Burson EC, et al. Effects of zinc propionate supplementation on growth performance, skeletal muscle fiber, and receptor characteristic in beef steers. J. Anim.Sci 2020;7:1–7.

77. Galyean ML, Malcolm-Callis KJ, Gunter SA, et al. Effect of zinc source and level and added copper lysine in the receiving diet on performance by growing and finishing steers. Prof Anim Sci 1995;11:139–48.

78. Spears J, Kegley E. Effect of zinc source (zinc oxide vs zinc proteinate) and level on performance, carcass characteristics, and immune response of growing and finishing steers. J Anim Sci 2002;80:2747–52.

79. Kegley EB, Silzell SA, Kreider DL, et al. The immune response and performance of calves supplemented with zinc from an organic and an inorganic source. Prof Anim Sci 2001;17:33–8.

80. Nunnery GA, Vasconcelos JT, Parsons CH, et al. Effect of source of supplemental zinc on performance and humoral immunity in beef heifers. J Anim Sci 2007;85:2304–13.

81. Rhoads AR, Stanton TL, Engle TE, et al. Effects of concentration and source of trace minerals on performance, immunity, mineral and lipid metabolism, and carcass characteristics of beef steers. Prof Anim Sci 2003;19:150–8.

82. Berrett CL, Wagner JJ, Neuhold KL, et al. Comparison of National Research Council standards and industry dietary trace mineral supplementation strategies for yearling feedlot steers. Prof Anim Sci 2015;3:237–47.

83. Lippy BA, Robison CA, Wilson BK. The effects of varying levels of trace mineral supplementation on performance, carcass characteristics, mineral balance, and antibody titer concentrations in feedlot cattle. Translational Anim. Sci. 2022;6:1–16.

84. Niedermayer EK, Genther-Schroeder ON, Loy DD, et al. Effect of varying trace mineral supplementation of steers with or without hormone implants on growth and carcass characteristics. J Anim Sci 2018;96:1159–70.

85. Zanetti D, Menezes ACB, Silva FAS, et al. In situ and in vitro estimation of mineral release from common feedstuffs. J Agri Sci 2017;155:1160–73.

86. Pogge DJ, Hansen SL. Supplemental vitamin C improves marbling in feedlot cattle consuming high sulfur diets. J Anim Sci 2013;91:4303–14.

87. Pyatt NA, Berger LL, Nash TG. Effects of vitamin A and restricted intake on performance, carcass characteristics, and serum retinol status in Angus × Simmental feedlot cattle. Prof Anim Sci 2005;21:318–31.

88. Gorocica-Buenfil MA, Fluharty FL, Reynolds CK, et al. Effect of dietary vitamin A concentration and roasted soybean inclusion on marbling, adipose cellularity, and fatty acid composition of beef. J Anim Sci 2007a;85:2230–42.

89. Gorocica-Buenfil MA, Fluharty FL, Reynolds CK, et al. Effect of dietary vitamin A restriction on marbling and conjugated linoleic acid content in Holstein steers. J Anim Sci 2007b;85:2243–55.

90. Gorocica-Buenfil MA, Fluharty FL, Bohn T, et al. Effect of low vitamin A diets with high-moisture or dry corn on marbling and adipose tissue fatty acid composition of beef steers. J Anim Sci 2007c;85:3355–66.

91. Gorocica-Buenfil MA, Fluharty FL, Loerch SC. Effect of vitamin A restriction on carcass characteristics and immune status of beef steers. J Anim Sci 2008;86:1609–16.

92. Bryant TC, Wagner JJ, Tatum JD, et al. Effect of dietary supplemental vitamin A concentration on performance, carcass merit, serum metabolites, and lipogenic enzyme activity in yearling beef steers. J Anim Sci 2010;88:1465–78.

Trace Mineral Nutrition of Sheep

Robert J. Van Saun, DVM, MS, PhD, DACT, DACVIM (Nutrition)

KEYWORDS

• Trace minerals • Sheep • Requirements • Mineral interactions • Supplementation

KEY POINTS

• Sheep have requirements for all trace elements; however, they are more sensitive to copper toxicosis than other ruminants requiring careful dietary formulation.
• Trace mineral requirements for sheep are mostly determined through factorial models accounting for maintenance, fleece production, pregnancy, growth, and lactation.
• Required amounts of trace elements need to account for availability of the element from various dietary sources and address geographic differences.
• Sheep copper nutrition is influenced by many dietary inhibitors affecting availability, primarily molybdenum, sulfur, iron, and zinc.

INTRODUCTION

Trace mineral biologic functions have been addressed elsewhere in this issue (see W. Swecker article on "Trace mineral function and requirements, content of common feeds, and assessment of the feeds, supplements, and animals") and other reviews.[1–3] Sheep are no different from other ruminant species in that they have a requirement for all the trace minerals, cobalt (Co), copper (Cu), iodine (I), iron (Fe), manganese (Mn), selenium (Se), and zinc (Zn).[4] What is unique relative to trace mineral nutritional management in sheep is their high sensitivity to Cu toxicosis.[1,5] This being stated, many published reports addressing sheep mineral nutrition describe challenges with Cu deficiency due to either inadequate dietary Cu or reduced Cu availability resultant of inhibitors.[6–9] The most described interactions are with Cu, sulfur (S), and molybdenum (Mo).[10–12] Additionally, consumed Fe can interfere with Cu availability.[1,13] Following Cu, Se nutrition poses the second most reported trace mineral issue with sheep.[1,14,15] This article will review sheep trace mineral requirements through the life cycle and address supplementation practices under various sheep management enterprises. A case study will be presented to highlight the diagnostic and nutritional intervention process.

Department of Veterinary and Biomedical Sciences, College of Agricultural Sciences, Pennsylvania State University, 108C Animal, Veterinary and Biomedical Sciences Building, University Park, PA 16802-3500, USA
E-mail address: rjv10@psu.edu

Vet Clin Food Anim 39 (2023) 517–533
https://doi.org/10.1016/j.cvfa.2023.07.001
0749-0720/23/© 2023 Elsevier Inc. All rights reserved.

TRACE MINERAL REQUIREMENTS

The most recent publication defining sheep requirements is the National Research Council (NRC) report published in 2007.[4] This report addresses all small ruminants, that is, sheep, goats, camelids, and cervids, in contrast to the previous NRC Nutrient Requirements of Sheep published in 1985.[16] In the 1985 publication, trace mineral requirements were exclusively based on dietary concentration recommendations, namely parts per million (ppm or milligram/kilogram) of dietary dry matter (DM). In the period between the 1985 and 2007 sheep nutrient requirement publications, tremendous changes occurred in genetics, productivity, and management practices.[17] During this same period, sheep numbers in the United States declined markedly, suggesting less emphasis on sheep nutritional research.[17] In spite of these limitations, the NRC (2007) report did provide a factorial methodology in predicting requirements for most of the trace minerals (**Table 1**).[4]

Cobalt

Dietary supplementation of Co is a unique nutritional requirement of ruminants. Dietary Co is used by rumen microbes to generate cyanocobalamin (eg, vitamin B_{12}) that can be absorbed in the small intestine by the host sheep. Microbes will generate both biologically active and inactive forms of vitamin B_{12}.[1] Prevailing rumen conditions (ie, ruminal acidosis) may adversely affect cyanocobalamin production. The sheep Co requirement is based on dietary content and recommended as 0.1 mg/kg dietary DM and this has not changed between the 1985 and 2007 reports.[4,16] Forage Co is low in many geographic regions, primarily Australia and New Zealand but also in the United States in Northeastern and Atlantic coast states, parts of Michigan and Iowa.[18,19]

Copper

The NRC (2007) report assumes an availability of dietary Cu to range between 4.5% (pasture and concentrates) and 6% (harvested forage) for adult sheep with variable availability for younger sheep (**Table 2**).[4] Higher Cu availability is observed from conserved forages compared with fresh pasture (**Fig. 1**). This difference in Cu availability is suggested to be related to inadvertent soil ingestion during pasture grazing and a consequence of high soil Fe content impacting Cu availability.[1] Plant Cu is associated with the chloroplast, vacuole, and cell wall as a component of various enzymes.[20] Binding of Cu with associated enzymes may limit availability in consuming fresh plant tissue during grazing; however, harvesting the forage may release Cu due to plant tissue degradation making the Cu more available. Dietary Zn through its induction of metallothionein synthesis in the enterocyte can reduce dietary Cu availability through the nonspecific binding with metallothionein and enterocyte sloughing.[3] A suggested ratio of 4:1 relative to dietary Zn-to-Cu is suggested to minimize this interaction. Other dietary factors such as Mo and S also are significant potential inhibitors of dietary Cu availability.

In the rumen, Mo and S can combine to form various molecular weight thiomolybdate compounds that bind to Cu, limiting availability or utilization if absorbed.[10,11,21] Depending on rumen fluid pH and dietary Mo and S content, monothiomolybdate ($MoSO_3$), dithiomolybdate (MoS_2O_2), trithiomolybdate (MoS_3O), and tetrathiomolybdate (MoS_4) compounds can form.[10] Typical rumen conditions where pH is less than 6.5 result in trithiomolybdate and tetrathiomolybdate forms predominating. These forms bind dietary Cu and prevent its absorption. Monothiomolybdate and dithiomolybdate forms are more common when the ratio of Mo:S is low (<10:1).[10] Lower

Table 1

Comparison of dietary trace mineral recommendations (mg/kg dietary dry matter) or factorial requirement models (milligram/day) for sheep based on the NRC publications[4,16]

Mineral	Report	Maintenance	Gestation	Lactation	Growth
Cobalt	1985	0.1			0.1
	2007	0.1			0.1
Copper	1985	8.0	8.0	8.0	10.0
	2007	$((0.004*BW_{kg}) + (0.0137*Fleece_{kg}))/AC$	$0.05*BirthWt_{kg}/AC$	$0.2*Milk_{kg}/AC$	$1.06*LWG/AC$
Iodine	1985	0.1	0.1	0.8	0.8
	2007	0.5	0.5	0.5	0.5
Iron	1985	30	40	40	50
	2007	$((0.014*BW_{kg}) + (0.082*Fleece_{kg}))/0.1$	$0.5*BirthWt_{kg}/0.1$	$0.9*Milk_{kg}/0.1$	$55*LWG/AC$
Manganese	1985	20	40	40	20
	2007	$((0.002*BW_{kg}) + (0.0068*Fleece_{kg}))/0.0075$	$0.02*BirthWt_{kg}/0.0075$	$0.055*Milk_{kg}/0.0075$	$0.47*LWG/0.0075$
Selenium	1985	0.3	0.3	0.3	0.3
	2007	$((0.00025*BW_{kg}) + (0.001*Fleece_{kg}))/AC$	$0.0025*BirthWt_{kg}/AC$	$0.14*Milk_{kg}/AC$	$0.5*LWG/AC$
Zinc	1985	20	33	33	33
	2007	$((0.076*BW_{kg}) + (0.315*Fleece_{kg}))/0.15$	$0.375*BirthWt_{kg}/0.15$	$7.4*Milk_{kg}/0.15$	$24*LWG/AC$

Abbreviations: AC, availability coefficient; Copper, 0; 06 for maintenance and pregnant ewes and 0, 045 for lactating ewes; Iron, 0; 5 preweaned lambs or 0, 19 weaned lambs; Selenium, 0; 31 forages and 0, 6 concentrates.

Table 2
Dietary absorption coefficients for copper and zinc for growing and adult sheep as defined by National Research Council 2007 publication[4]

Animal Class and Weight Class	Absorption Coefficient	
	Copper	Zinc
Lamb, preweaning		
5 kg BW	0.90	0.55
10 kg BW	0.53	0.55
20 kg BW	0.20	0.30
Lamb postweaning, pasture	0.045	0.20
Lamb postweaning, feedlot	0.060	0.20
Ewe, gestation	0.060	0.15
Ewe, lactation	0.045	0.15

molecular weight thiomolybdates may be absorbed and potentially can bind to Cu in proteins altering biologic function.[10,22]

A dietary ratio of 6 to 8:1 for Cu-to-Mo is recommended for sheep to maintain adequate Cu availability. Dietary Cu:Mo ratio below 4:1 will induce reduced Cu availability with lower ratios being consistent with induced Cu deficiency. Ratios above 12 to 16:1 would be suggestive of potential Cu toxicosis. The NRC Cu requirements and defined Cu bioavailability assume dietary Mo being less than 1 ppm. Dietary Cu concentrations for various life stages are similar to previous recommendations and range between 5.5 and 12 mg/kg DM (**Fig. 2**).[4] An upper intake amount of 24 mg Cu or 15 mg/kg dietary DM is suggested, although this will need to be adjusted relative to presence of inhibitors.[4] Diets with higher Mo, S, or both need to address potential lower Cu availability (see **Fig. 1**). Sulfur alone can reduce dietary Cu availability through the formation of copper sulfide an insoluble Cu compound.[23] Dietary S forms such as sulfates are reduced to sulfide, which can bind to most cations forming insoluble forms.

Iodine

The primary role for I is in support of thyroid-generated hormones that influence cellular metabolism and basal metabolic rate. Iodine is efficiently absorbed by the thyroid gland and accounts for 80% of body I.[1] Goitrogens are compounds that interfere

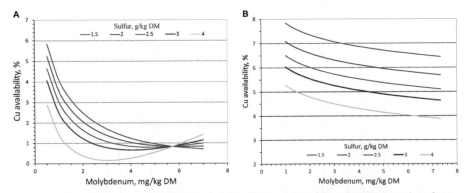

Fig. 1. Predicted dietary copper (Cu) availability from pasture (A) or hay (B) based on forage molybdenum and sulfur concentrations. Redrawn from the equations presented in Suttle, 2010.[1]

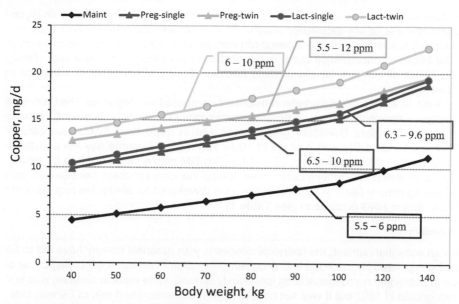

Fig. 2. NRC (2007) recommended copper intake (milligram/day) relative to body weight and physiologic status of maintenance (Maint), pregnancy (Preg), and lactation (Lact) with single or twin fetuses.[4]

with either I uptake or thyroid hormone synthesis.[1,2] Selenium-dependent 5'-deiodinase enzymes (Types I, II, and III) are responsible for converting thyroxin (T_4) into the active thyroid hormone triiodothyronine (T_3).[24] Many regions of the world are considered I-deficient in soil and forages.[2] In the United States, geographic regions around the Great Lakes and Pacific Northwest have potential I deficiency from forage and water.[4] Dietary recommendations for I requirements range from 0.1 to 1.25 mg/kg DM in various publications. Diets with goitrogens are suggested to have increased I at 2.0 mg/kg DM. Dietary I concentration recommendations for sheep were increased from 1985 recommendations to 0.5 mg/kg DM for maintenance, gestation, and growth and 0.8 mg/kg DM for lactating sheep.[4]

Iron

Iron has many biologic roles in heme compounds (ie, hemoglobin, myoglobin, and cytochromes), Fe–S complexes associated with electron transfer, and other nonheme enzymes (ie, aconitase, pyruvate kinase, and various hydroxylases).[1,2] Other than issues with internal parasites, Fe generally is not a deficiency problem but more of an excess issue that may interfere with availability of other minerals. Excess Fe can originate from dietary ingredients, water, or a combination. Excess dietary Fe can act as a prooxidant. Sheep Fe requirements were changed from a dietary concentration recommendation to a factorial model approach, although no recommendation model for growth was provided (see **Table 1**).[4] Using the factorial requirement models, dietary Fe concentration would generally be lower than previous recommendations, although this varies by body weight and life stage.

Manganese

Most metabolic reactions associated with carbohydrates, lipids, and cholesterol are influenced by Mn-dependent enzymes. Mucopolysaccharide matrix and chondroitin sulfate side chains as structural components of bone and cartilage depend on glyco-syltransferase, a Mn-dependent enzyme.[1,2] Superoxide dismutase within the mito-chondria is Mn-dependent. Placental Mn transfer is limited as evidenced by minimal fetal hepatic concentration but it is concentrated in colostrum.[25] Generally, dietary Mn is not of concern for sheep diets because forage Mn content is adequate in most regions.

Grass forages contain a greater Mn content compared with legumes. The Dairy One Forage Laboratory library (https://apps.dairyone.com/feedcomposition/) reports mean (± Standard Deviation) grass forage Mn in more than 60,000 samples of 87.7 ± 67 mg/kg DM with a range of 20 to 155 mg/kg. Legume hay Mn content in more than 42,000 samples was 39 ± 18 mg/kg DM with a range of 20 to 57 mg/kg. Previous sheep Mn requirements were based on concentration between 20 and 40 mg/kg dietary DM.[16] A factorial model was developed for sheep Mn requirements in the recent NRC publication (see **Table 1**).[4]

Selenium

As an essential nutrient, the historical concerns with potential toxicity have led to Se being regulated by the Food and Drug Administration.[26] An essential biologic role of Se in nutritional myodegeneration (previously termed white muscle disease) was first recognized in 1957 but it was not until 1972 that the antioxidant role of Se was iden-tified through its role in glutathione peroxidase.[27] Additional selenoproteins have been recognized including thioredoxin reductase, iodothyronine 5'deiodinases, and seleno-proteins P and W.[1] Selenium's interaction with vitamin E in their interconnected roles as cellular antioxidants have been well recognized. Most regions of the United States and elsewhere in the world forage Se content is inadequate to meet animal needs either due to low soil Se content or soil conditions that restrict plant Se uptake (ie, acid pH, Fe, and aluminum content).[27] The US Great Plains states from Montana and North Dakota south to New Mexico have sporadic areas of high soil Se content coupled with alkaline pH facilitating plant Se content or Se-accumulating plants that can potentially cause chronic or acute toxicosis, respectively, when consumed.[27,28]

Sheep Se requirement has been reported to be between 0.05 and 0.15 mg/kg die-tary DM; however, 0.3 mg/kg dietary DM is often recommended.[16] Inorganic Se sour-ces such as sodium selenite and selenate are subject to rumen microbial alteration making the Se unavailable and dietary S content can compete for intestinal absorp-tion.[27,29] Current regulations allow dietary Se supplementation at a level of 0.3 mg/kg of total diet. Daily supplemental Se for sheep is 0.7 mg. Since 2000, an organic Se form, namely selenomethionine has been approved for use in the United States at the same supplementation rate. In Europe, inorganic Se sources are allowed to be supplemented at 0.5 mg/kg, whereas selenomethionine is restricted to no more than 0.2 mg/kg due to its greater bioavailability and potential human health risk.[30] Weekly dosing of selenite or selenomethionine in sheep at 0.3, 0.9, and 1.5 mg/kg di-etary DM showed much greater Se status, measured as whole blood Se concentra-tion, and a linear increase with increasing dosing for selenomethionine, whereas there was no difference in Se status between 0.9 and 1.5 mg/kg from inorganic Se.[14] Benefits of supranutritional Se supplementation on immunologic function and animal health has been recognized.[31–35] Maximum tolerable level for Se in nonrumi-nants is 2 mg/kg, whereas it is 5 mg/kg for ruminants.[36]

Zinc

More than 200 different enzymes have their activity associated with Zn.[1,2] Zinc is asso-ciated with cell differentiation and proliferation resultant of its associated in RNA and

DNA polymerases. Zinc-metalloenzymes influence vitamin A, carbohydrate, and lipid metabolism and male and female reproduction. Loss of taste and smell and reduced growth are considered early signs of Zn deficiency. Skin and its appendages are sensitive to Zn status leading to classic deficiency disease of parakeratosis, although hyperkeratosis and altered hair, fleece, or hooves are also affected.[1] Plant oxalates and phytate as well as Cu, calcium, and Fe can reduce Zn availability. A forage nutrient content survey from central and western United States region reported more than 75% of forages contained inadequate Zn.[37] Reviewing the forage database from Dairy One Laboratory mean ($\pm$ Standard Deviation) Zn content was 24 $\pm$ 13 mg/kg (range: 11–37 mg/kg; n = 42,448) and 28 $\pm$ 23 mg/kg (4.5–51 mg/kg; n = 29,429) for legume and grass forages, respectively.

Dietary sheep Zn recommendations from the NRC (1985) publication ranged between 20 and 33 mg/kg dietary DM.[16] The factorial models estimating Zn requirements in the NRC (2007) publication have increased Zn requirement.[4] Maintenance Zn requirement using the factorial model would suggest a dietary Zn concentration of 40 to 45 mg/kg, essentially doubling the previous recommendation. This new requirement would suggest forages would not be able to provide sufficient Zn without additional supplementation. Absorption coefficient for dietary Zn is 0.15 for adults and higher for younger sheep (see **Table 2**).

ESTABLISHING TRACE MINERAL NEEDS FOR THE FLOCK

A repeated concept throughout this issue is focusing on the differences in trace mineral status by geographic region. As much as owners wish for some simple solution of "what is the best mineral supplement," trace mineral supplementation needs to be focused on forage trace mineral status, which is a function of the geographic region.

Forage Mineral Testing

A representative sample(s) of forage(s) being fed needs to be collected and submitted to an accredited forage testing laboratory. A description of forage sample collection can be found on the National Forage Testing Association website (www. foragetesting.org). A grab sample is not an appropriate sampling method. One should use a forage probe (https://www.foragetesting.org/hay-probes) to collect through the baled forage layers. Depending on forage bale size, 2-to-3 core samples should be obtained from each bale. Approximately 10% to 20% of the forage inventory should be sampled. Total collected sample should be mixed thoroughly, quartered, and opposing quarters combined for submission. A total of 100 to 150 g of sample (ie, pint-sized ziplock bag) submitted to the laboratory. Submitting too much material results in the laboratory having to subsample the submission, which may skew results.

Sampling wet forages is more challenging, especially that of pasture. Silages should be collected by sampling across the silage bunk face. Ideally have material taken from the entire silage face and mixed. A subsample of the mixed material can be collected by the quartering system, placed in an airtight bag with air expelled, and frozen. The sample should be sent frozen and on ice to the laboratory. Pasture sampling can be attempted through an observational selective harvesting method mimicking what the animals are eating, or by a random ring toss in the pasture harvesting plant material within the ring. Due to their moisture content, pasture samples should be frozen and submitted frozen to the laboratory.

Most accredited forage laboratories will perform wet chemistry analysis for minerals because near infrared spectroscopy methods are inappropriate to accurately determine feed mineral content.[38]

Wet chemistry methods are typically performed with intercoupled plasma spectroscopy (ICP) with atomic emission or mass spectroscopy. Trace minerals commonly determined by most laboratories are Fe, Mn, Cu, and Zn. Sulfur and Mo are often additional cost options but these should be determined due to their potential for interfering with Cu availability. Some laboratories will perform feed Se analysis; however, this is a much higher cost item. Determination of forage Se will depend on the geographic region where there is potential for higher Se content. Geographic areas known to be Se deficient would preclude performing this expensive test unless there is some potential concern.

Feed Label Interpretation

Commercial concentrate products and mineral supplements are required to meet State-defined product label requirements. The American Association of Feed Control Officials publishes a "Model Bill" defining feed labeling rules that most States will adopt or modify for their feed label regulations.[39] Two required feed label components include the guaranteed analysis and ingredient listing. The guaranteed analysis provides limited compositional analysis of the product on an "as fed" basis. These values are reported as minimums, maximums, or both depending on nutrient. State feed regulations dictate what nutrient values are required on a feed label and this is species specific. Most states require Cu composition (minimum and maximum) for sheep products. Although guaranteed analysis information is of some use, laboratory analysis of a representative sample would be preferred.

The ingredient listing on a product label presents the product ingredients on a highest to lowest incorporation rate on an as-fed basis.[39] The ingredient listing provides an opportunity to evaluate mineral sources used. Minerals may be inorganic, organic, or a combination sources. Copper oxide as a mineral source is considered unavailable for ruminants.[40] This is in contrast to Cu oxide wire particles (discussed below). Many sheep products contain sodium molybdate but Mo content is not a required parameter for the guaranteed analysis. Commercial supplement and mineral products should be laboratory analyzed to provide a more comprehensive mineral profile of the product.

Diagnostic Testing

Blood testing and tissue, primarily liver, mineral concentrations can be reasonably used to evaluate nutritive status of the animal (see W. Swecker article on "Trace mineral function and requirements, content of common feeds, and assessment of the feeds, supplements, and animals").[41–44] Hepatic mineral concentrations represent the primary storage pool of trace minerals and are most sensitive to nutritive status.[41,44] Interpretation can be challenging because many laboratories do not have sufficiently robust reference criteria for sheep of various ages (**Table 3**).

Use of serum, plasma, or whole blood is often the collected sample in assessing nutritive status because this is the most convenient sample (see **Table 3**). Applicability of blood samples for assessing nutritive status depends on the trace mineral.[41–43] Either serum or whole blood concentrations as good indicators of Se status, although serum is a more acute indicator of Se status compared with whole blood but prone to errors with a hemolyzed sample. Direct measures of serum Co, I, Mn, and Mo concentrations have only become available with the application of ICP/mass spectroscopy methods.[45] Serum Fe concentrations are useful but should be considered in combination with total Fe-binding capacity, ferritin, and percent transferrin saturation measures. Serum Cu and Zn concentrations have somewhat limited diagnostic value on an individual basis, except for extreme high or low concentrations. Collection of multiple samples (n = 10–15) accounting for individual variation has been shown to

Table 3
Suggested hepatic (microgram/gram dry weight) and serum trace mineral concentrations for healthy adult sheep

Trace Mineral	Hepatic	Serum
Cobalt	0.08–0.35	0.18–2.0 ng/mL
Copper	72–475	0.70–1.7 μg/mL
Iron	250–4000	1.2–2.20 μg/mL
Manganese	4.6–21	1.0–6.0 ng/mL
Molybdenum	0.3–4.7	1.0–5.0 ng/mL
Selenium	0.8–6.1	110–160 ng/mL
Selenium, whole blood		120–350 ng/mL
Zinc	80–460	0.8–1.2 μg/mL

improve diagnostic value of serum mineral concentrations.[42] Mineral analysis for this many samples becomes cost prohibitive, especially for smaller flocks. Use of pooled samples might help to reduce costs yet maintain a level of flock diagnostic value.[46]

TRACE MINERAL MANAGEMENT METHODS

Should a trace mineral toxicosis be recognized (see John Buchweitz and colleagues, "Trace mineral toxicosis in ruminants" in this issue), the offending source or sources of the mineral in question need to be removed from the diet. A primary concern with sheep is Cu toxicosis because compared with other ruminants, sheep have a lesser ability to excrete Cu resulting in liver accumulation.[1,5] Dietary administration of interfering minerals such as Mo and S alone will not reduce hepatic Cu content.[5] All sources of Cu in the diet need to be removed or reduced to induce a Cu deficient diet as well as adding Cu interfering sources such as calcium sulfate, molybdenum sulfate, or sodium sulfate.[23,47] In situations of trace mineral deficiency, a source of the deficient mineral or minerals needs to be provided. Response to supplementation depends on method (eg, oral or parenteral), modality (**Box 1**), and frequency.

Free Choice Trace Mineral Salt

By-and-far providing trace minerals through the provision of a salt-based trace mineral product is the most common method in most sheep operations. This is the least labor-intensive method; however, it is also fraught with challenges resulting from individual

---

Box 1
Methods of trace mineral supplementation

- Soluble mineral sources dissolved in water source
- Bolus or drenching
- Free-choice trace mineralized salt supplement
- Direct incorporation into diet as TMR
- Top-dress on diet
- Incorporated into a concentrate supplement
- Slow-release rumen boluses
- Parenteral injection

variation in salt consumption.[48] Animals, including sheep, only have an appetite for ingestion of sodium, thus the use of salt to control intake. The higher the salt content of the mineral, the lower the intake. The FDA allows for a maximum of 90 mg/kg Se in a free choice mineral. This assumes greater than 90% salt and an intake of 0.25 to 0.33 ounces per day or delivery of 0.7 mg Se per day. Copper content of a sheep trace mineral salt is recommended to be less than 30 mg/kg compared with goat and cattle salts containing greater than 300 mg/kg Cu. Many commercial sheep mineral products have less Se content as the feed label indicates a much higher intake rate. One should directly average intake of the mineral supplement to properly assess mineral supplementation adequacy. Under range conditions mineral can be supplied once or more per week rather than a daily delivery. There is interest in individual mineral feeding allowing the animal "to choose" what is needed. These "cafeteria mineral" feeding programs have not been shown to adequately supplement minerals according to animal needs as the animals has no "nutritional knowledge" beyond an appetite for sodium.[49–51]

Dietary Incorporation

This supplementation approach might be considered the "gold standard" of trace mineral supplementation. In this approach, the diet is formulated for the appropriate balance of trace minerals, hopefully addressing interfering elements, and supplied daily as the trace mineral sources (often a premix) is directly incorporated into a total mixed ration (TMR). Dietary incorporation ensures a more consistent intake rate. Another option is to provide a "complete" supplement that consists of energy and protein sources as well as mineral and vitamins as a concentrate to complement the forage program. This is most often the approach for many sheep operations. Amount of concentrate fed can be titrated to nutrient need based on life cycle stage.

Slow-Release Boluses

In Australia and New Zealand where sheep production is predominately pasture-based, the prevailing soil conditions result in forage trace mineral deficiencies in Co, Cu, Se, and Zn.[19,52] For animals being managed on large pastures slow-release boluses have been used to address the trace mineral deficiency issues.[6,8,9,53] These boluses provide elemental Cu^{++} as the Cu oxide wire particles are degraded by the low pH of the abomasum. Their effect is up to 6 months and excessive administration can result in Cu toxicity.[54] The author has used 2 g Cu oxide wire particle boluses in grazing sheep to maintain Cu status in the face of excess forage Mo (Van Saun, unpublished data 2016).

Parenteral Injection

Two trace minerals, Cu and Se, have been the primary ones where a commercial injectable product has been available for use in sheep. Parenteral Cu injection originally was using either Cu glycine or Cu-complex with calcium ethylenediamine tetra-acetic acid (EDTA). Copper glycine subcutaneous injection induces a necrotic lesion at the injection site and was recommended to be injected ventrally in the brisket region.[55] Similarly, intramuscular injection of Cu-EDTA induced severe swelling and had variable effects on hepatic Cu concentration.[55] Currently in the United Kingdom, Australia, and New Zealand, there is a parenteral Cu-methionate product that is administered intramuscularly at a dose of 20 mg Cu per kg body weight. Sodium selenite injection has been a mainstay product in sheep production in geographic regions of Se deficiency. Commercial parenteral Se products will have vitamin E as an antioxidant but this is not at a level sufficient enough to provide supplemental vitamin E.

Products have varying Se concentrations dosage to allow for differing volumes of administration for a given animal. Parenteral Se supplementation in Se-deficient beef heifers showed rapid urinary excretion and return to low blood Se concentrations within 28 days.[56]

More recently, a multiple mineral parenteral product has been introduced into the US market. This sheep product contains Mn (10 mg/mL), Se (3 mg/mL), and Zn (40 mg/mL) without or with Cu (10 mg/mL); all minerals bound to EDTA, except Se. One study showed improved marking rate and lamb performance.[57] One must assess Cu status before administering any parenteral Cu solution.

Other Options

Weekly drenching of sheep with a week's equivalent of Se supplement source showed improved Se status compared with untreated control ewes.[14] This option is labor intensive and requires multiple animal handling times. Selenium fertilization can increase organic Se form in forages and improve Se nutritive status during the grazing season.[58,59] Forage Se fertilization is used in many countries outside the United States but it is allowed exclusively in the State of Oregon.

CASE STUDY

A commercial Finn, Dorset, Suffolk, and crossbred sheep flock (n = 250) was experiencing high lamb losses ranging from 17% to 25% as stillborn or early neonatal deaths. Approximately 6 years earlier, an adult ewe was diagnosed with Cu deficiency and associated spinal nerve demyelination along with lambs with enzootic ataxia (eg, swayback). The flock was not pastured and fed in confinement using a TMR. The diet consisted of purchased locally grown forages with some concentrate and a mineral premix. Forage base was mostly corn silage with corn fodder, clover, or alfalfa hay to provide dietary fiber, protein, or both. Nutritionists were unable to help the flock correct the problem with dietary modifications.

Diagnostic Testing

In communicating with the flock owner, arrangements were made for submission of lambs or ewes for necropsy or liver samples for mineral analyses to assess the flock's mineral status (**Table 4**). No microbiologic or other cause for ewe and lamb deaths was identified on necropsy. Additionally, forage samples were collected over time for nutrient testing (**Table 5**). Water analysis reports were provided, and these showed high Fe (8.25 and 3.84 mg/L; reference < 0.3 mg/L) and moderate S as sulfate (433 and 432 mg/L; reference <500 mg/L) content. From these data, Cu deficiency was

Table 4
Hepatic copper (Cu) and molybdenum (Mo) concentrations (microgram/gram dry weight) for affected lambs and ewes submitted for necropsy

Mineral	Lambs, n = 4	Ewes, n = 3
Copper	36.3 ± 16.7	18 ± 13.1
Molybdenum	1.9 ± 0.6	3.3 ± 1.6
Cu Reference	75–475	60–300
Mo Reference	1.5–3.0	

Data adapted from Herdt and Hoff, 2013, Michigan State University Nutrition Laboratory, and Van Saun, unpublished data.

Table 5
Forage copper (Cu), molybdenum (Mo) concentration (milligram/kg dry matter) and their ratio in forages from a sheep farm experiencing clinical signs of Cu deficiency

Forage Crop	Year	Copper	Molybdenum	Cu:Mo Ratio
Clover hay	2011	5.1	2.52	2.02
Corn silage	2011	14.8	0.51	29.0
Clover hay	2011	9.8	5.04	1.9
Corn silage	2012	6.6	5.48	1.2
Oatlage	2012	7.4	5.31	1.39
Corn silage	2013	7.0	5.33	1.31
Oat forage	2013	7.0	5.77	1.21
Clover silage	2014	14.8	1.5	9.87
Clover hay	2015	12.5	8.43	1.48
Corn fodder	2015	6.5	2.97	2.19
Corn silage	2015	3.6	7.15	0.50
Corn silage	2015	4.3	6.87	0.63
Oat baleage	2015	8.4	2.47	3.40
Clover hay	2016	12.5	8.43	1.48
Corn fodder	2016	6.5	2.97	2.19
Clover stubble	2017	10.8	1.72	6.27
Alfalfa hay	2018	9.2	1.7	5.41
Corn silage	2019	6.2	1.43	4.33
Corn silage	2020	5.5	4.81	1.14
Clover hay	2020	5.5	13.1	0.42

confirmed based on hepatic Cu concentration. Forage nutrient analysis monitoring showed consistently elevated Mo over time with all but 3 forages having a low Cu:Mo ratio (<5:1) indicative of inducing Cu deficiency. Alternative forage options were not available, thus dietary Cu availability needed to be corrected.

Dietary Evaluation and Correction

In evaluating the TMR for the flock as it was currently formulated, all macronutrients were adequately provided to meet the sheep needs depending on physiologic state. The flock TMR consisted of corn silage, dry forage, and a custom mineral-vitamin premix. Additional corn grain and soybean meal were added to adjust energy and protein for changing physiologic status of the flock. Trace minerals were supplied to meet requirements in the formulation but availability of Cu relative to interfering minerals was not considered. The Cu, S, and Mo content of the original TMR was 18 ppm, 0.21%, and 5.3 ppm, respectively. The custom mineral-vitamin premix was reformulated to increase Cu content to 480 ppm to account for the forage Mo and have an 8:1 Cu:Mo ratio in the TMR. The formulated intake of the premix was 0.18 lb mixed with 0.29 lb distillers' grains. This was the same incorporation rate for the original TMR. Analysis of the TMR showed between 38 and 43 ppm Cu and between 5.3 and 5.8 ppm Mo. Special arrangements were made with the feed company to produce a product for sheep with this high Cu content. The Cu content of the premix was modified on a yearly basis to account for any forage Mo changes. Diets were formulated for maintenance, early and late gestation, and lactation with this approach.

Table 6
Hepatic mineral concentrations (microgram/gram dry weight) for stillborn or deceased neonatal lambs from a sheep flock suspected of copper toxicity

Selenium (µg/g)	Cobalt (µg/g)	Copper (µg/g)	Iron (µg/g)	Manganese (µg/g)	Molybdenum (µg/g)	Zinc (µg/g)
3.4	0.13	135	405	21.1	1.1	502
2.4	0.08	40	394	15.9	1.1	327
1.4	0.12	13	509	17.6	1.8	314
1.4	0.06	53	657	6.9	2.2	320
1.1	0.04	39	404	6	2.6	385
1.2	0.18	12	266	6.2	4.2	199
2.6	0.51	33	813	14.7	1.5	299
1.4	0.13	9	258	8	4.3	106
1.5	0.1	35	310	13.6	3.8	356
1.6	0.05	53	398	13.1	4.4	481
2.5	0.15	136	250	23.6	2.7	513
3.7	0.17	200	886	44.8	2.5	609
3.3	0.07	94	432	11.6	1.3	222
Laboratory Reference Range						
1.0–2.5	0.3–0.6	75–300	200–600	6.0–12.0	1.5–3.0	60–270

Case Outcome and Recommendations

The first lambing season in which the additional dietary Cu was provided resulted in greatly improved lamb health and survival. Lamb losses were reduced to less than 2% compared with the previous 17% to 25%. During the second lambing season with dietary Cu supplementation, the flock owner reported a 50% lamb loss rate for early lambing ewes. A concern of potential Cu toxicosis was considered. Liver samples harvested from deceased lambs were submitted for mineral analysis (**Table 6**). Surprisingly, interpretation of hepatic Cu indicated ongoing Cu deficiency. Of the 13 samples, 4 were within the laboratory reference range; however, 3 of these lambs had been treated with a multimineral parenteral product before death. A review of the diet determined a new alfalfa hay had been incorporated into the TMR without earlier review or evaluation. Subsequent analysis showed this alfalfa hay to contain 15.4 ppm Cu and 22.1 ppm Mo. This test was repeated twice and sent to a second laboratory for confirmation. On removal of this forage, subsequent ewe and lamb health and survival improved. Although not all consider Mo directly inducing disease, this situation does suggest a situation of molybdenosis with secondary Cu deficiency.[60] The case study addresses the complexity of ruminant Cu nutrition and underscores the need to be cognizant of changing mineral content with feed ingredients requiring ongoing monitoring.

CLINICS CARE POINTS

- A dietary copper-to-molybdenum ratio of 6 to 8:1 is recommended to ensure adequate copper availability.
- Sulfur in combination with molybdenum, or independently, can inhibit copper availability; however, this mechanism can be used to address copper toxicity by increasing dietary sulfur content.

- Trace mineralized salt for sheep should contain less than 30 ppm copper and up to 90 ppm selenium.
- Direct dietary incorporation of trace mineral sources is more physiologic and ensures a more consistent intake.
- Free choice trace mineralized salt is a convenient method of providing needed trace minerals; however, individual intake is highly variable, expected intakes differ by salt content, and mineral sources vary in their availability all potentially leading to trace mineral issues.

DISCLOSURE

Grant funding received from Pennsylvania Department of Agriculture, American Dairy Goat Association, Zoetis.

REFERENCES

1. Suttle NF. Mineral nutrition of livestock. 4th edition. Oxfordshire, UK: CABI International; 2010.
2. McDowell LR. Minerals in animal and human nutrition. San Diego: Academic Press Inc; 1992.
3. Goff JP. Invited review: Mineral absorption mechanisms, mineral interactions that affect acid-base and antioxidant status, and diet considerations to improve mineral status. J Dairy Sci 2018;101:2763–813.
4. National Research Council. Nutrient requirements of small ruminants: sheep, goats, cervids, and new world camelids. Washington, DC: The National Academies Press; 2007.
5. Hidiroglou M, Heaney D, Hartin K. Copper poisoning in a flock of sheep. Copper excretion patterns after treatment with molybdenum and sulfur or penicillamine. Can Vet J 1984;25:377.
6. Judson G, Trengove C, Langman M, et al. Copper supplementation of sheep. Aust Vet J 1984;61:40–3.
7. Suttle N. Effectiveness of orally administered cupric oxide needles in alleviating hypocupraemia in sheep and cattle. Vet Rec 1981;108:417–20.
8. Whitelaw A, Fawcett A, MacDonald A. Cupric oxide needles in the prevention of swayback. Vet Rec 1982;110:522.
9. Judson G, Brown T, Gray D, et al. Oxidized copper wire particles for copper therapy in sheep. Aust J Agric Res 1982;33:1073–83.
10. Gould L, Kendall NR. Role of the rumen in copper and thiomolybdate absorption. Nutr Res Rev 2011;24:176–82.
11. Smith B, Wright H. Copper: Molybdenum interaction: Effect of dietary molybdenum on the binding of copper to plasma proteins in sheep. J Comp Pathol 1975;85:299–305.
12. Suttle N. The interactions between copper, molybdenum, and sulphur in ruminant nutrition. Annu Rev Nutr 1991;11:121–40.
13. de Sousa IK, Hamad Minervino AH, Sousa Rdos S, et al. Copper deficiency in sheep with high liver iron accumulation. Vet Med Int 2012;2012:207950.
14. Hall JA, Van Saun RJ, Bobe G, et al. Organic and inorganic selenium: I. Oral bioavailability in ewes. J Anim Sci 2012;90:568–76.
15. Stewart WC, Bobe G, Vorachek WR, et al. Organic and inorganic selenium: II. Transfer efficiency from ewes to lambs. J Anim Sci 2012;90:577–84.

16. National Research Council. Nutrient requirements of sheep. 6th revised edition. San Diego: National Academies Press; 1985.
17. National Research Council. Changes in the sheep industry in the United States: making the transition from tradition. San Diego: National Academies Press; 2008.
18. Ammerman C. Recent developments in cobalt and copper in ruminant nutrition: A review. J Dairy Sci 1970;53:1097–107.
19. Lee J, Masters D, Judson G, et al. Current issues in trace element nutrition of grazing livestock in Australia and New Zealand. Aust J Agric Res 1999;50: 1341–64.
20. Burkhead JL, Gogolin Reynolds KA, Abdel-Ghany SE, et al. Copper homeostasis. New Phytol 2009;182:799–816.
21. Suttle NF. Recent studies of the copper-molybdenum antagonism. Proc Nutr Soc 1974;33:299–305.
22. Dick AT, Dewey DW, Gawthorne JM. Thiomolybdates and the copper–molybdenum–sulphur interaction in ruminant nutrition. J Agric Sci 2009;85:567–8.
23. Suttle NF. Control of hepatic copper retention in Texel ram lambs by dietary supplementation with copper antagonists followed by a copper depletion regimen. Anim Feed Sci Technol 2012;173:194–200.
24. Arthur JR, Nicol F, Beckett GJ. The role of selenium in thyroid hormone metabolism and effects of selenium deficiency on thyroid hormone and iodine metabolism. Biol Trace Elem Res 1992;33:37–42.
25. Van Saun R. Mineral and Vitamin Deficiencies in Aborted and Stillborn Calves. In: Szenci O, Mee J, Bleul U, et al, editors. Bovine Prenatal, Perinatal and neonatal medicine. 1st edition. Budapest, Hungary: Hungarian Association for Buiatrics; 2021. p. 246–60.
26. James L, Panter K, Mayland H, et al. Selenium poisoning in livestock: A review and progress. Selenium in Agriculture and the Environment 1989;23:123–31.
27. National Research Council. Selenium in nutrition: revised edition. Washington, D.C.: National Academies Press; 1983.
28. Mayland H, Gough L, Stewart K. Selenium mobility in soils and its absorption, translocation, and metabolism in plants. 1990 Billings Land Reclaimation Symposium 1991;55-64.
29. Galbraith ML, Vorachek WR, Estill CT, et al. Rumen Microorganisms Decrease Bioavailability of Inorganic Selenium Supplements. Biol Trace Elem Res 2016; 171:338–43.
30. Standing Committee on the Food Chain and Animal Health. Commission implementing regulation (EU) No 427/2013 of 8 may 2013. Brussels, Belgium: Official Journal of the European Union; 2013. L127/L120-122.
31. Kiremidjian-Schumacher L, Roy M, Wishe H, et al. Regulation of cellular immune responses by selenium. Biol Trace Elem Res 1992;33:23–35.
32. Hall JA, Bobe G, Vorachek WR, et al. Effect of supranutritional maternal and colostral selenium supplementation on passive absorption of immunoglobulin G in selenium-replete dairy calves. J Dairy Sci 2014;97:4379–91.
33. Hall JA, Isaiah A, McNett ERL, et al. Supranutritional Selenium-Yeast Supplementation of Beef Cows during the Last Trimester of Pregnancy Results in Higher Whole-Blood Selenium Concentrations in Their Calves at Weaning, but Not Enough to Improve Nasal Microbial Diversity. Animals (Basel) 2022;12.
34. Hall JA, Vorachek WR, Stewart WC, et al. Selenium supplementation restores innate and humoral immune responses in footrot-affected sheep. PLoS One 2013;8:e82572.

35. Stewart WC, Bobe G, Pirelli GJ, et al. Organic and inorganic selenium: III. Ewe and progeny performance. J Anim Sci 2012;90:4536–43.
36. National Research Council. Mineral tolerance of animals: 2005. San Diego: National Academies Press; 2006.
37. Mortimer R, Dargatz D, Corah L. Forage analyses from cow-calf herds in 23 states in: USDA:APHIS:vs. Fort Collins, CO: Centers for Epidemiology and Animal Health; 1999. p. 31.
38. Jones G, Wade NS, Baker JP, et al. Use of near infrared reflectance spectroscopy in forage testing. J Dairy Sci 1987;70:1086–91.
39. AAFCO. AAFCO official publication. Champaign, IL: American Association of Feed Control Officials; 2023.
40. Langlands J, Donald G, Bowles J, et al. Trace Element Nutrition of Grazing Animals. III. Copper Oxide Powder as a Copper Supplement. Aust J Agric Res 1989;40:187–93.
41. Ensley S. Evaluating Mineral Status in Ruminant Livestock. Vet Clin North Am Food Anim Pract 2020;36:525–46.
42. Herdt TH, Hoff B. The use of blood analysis to evaluate trace mineral status in ruminant livestock. Vet Clin North Am Food Anim Pract 2011;27:255–83.
43. Herdt TH, Rumbeiha W, Braselton WE. The Use of Blood Analyses to Evaluate Mineral Status in Livestock. Vet Clin North Am Food Anim Pract 2000;16:423–44.
44. Suttle N. Problems in the Diagnosis and Anticipation of Trace Mineral Deficiencies in Grazing Livestock. Vet Rec 1986;119:148–52.
45. Radke SL, Ensley SM, Hansen SL. Inductively coupled plasma mass spectrometry determination of hepatic copper, manganese, selenium, and zinc concentrations in relation to sample amount and storage duration. J Vet Diagn Invest 2020; 32:103–7.
46. Humann-Ziehank E, Tegtmeyer PC, Seelig B, et al. Variation of serum selenium concentrations in German sheep flocks and implications for herd health management consultancy. Acta Vet Scand 2013;55:1–8.
47. Wells NH, Hallford DM, Hernandez JA, et al. Case Report - Use of Calcium Sulfate to Alleviate Signs of Copper Toxicosis in Ewe Lambs. Bov Pract 2001; 35:70–2.
48. Tait R, Fisher L. Variability in individual animal's intake of minerals offered free-choice to grazing ruminants. Anim Feed Sci Technol 1996;62:69–76.
49. Pamp D., Goodrich R., Meiske J., Free-choice selection of minerals by lambs. J Anim Sci 1975;41(1):413 Abstract.
50. Pamp D, Goodrich R, Meiske J. Review of the practice of feeding minerals free choice. World Review of Animal Production 1976;12:13.
51. Muller LD, Schaffer LV, Ham LC, et al. Cafeteria style free-choice mineral feeder for lactating dairy cows. J Dairy Sci 1977;60:1574–82.
52. Grace ND, Knowles SO. Trace element supplementation of livestock in new zealand: meeting the challenges of free-range grazing systems. Vet Med Int 2012; 2012:639472.
53. Judson GJ, Vandergraaff R, Inglis SW, et al. Oxidized copper wire particles as an oral copper supplement in sheep. Agricutural Record 1983;10:12–4.
54. Hamar DW, Bedwell CL, Johnson JL, et al. Iatrogenic copper toxicosis induced by administering copper oxide boluses to neonatal calves. J Vet Diagn Invest 1997;9:441–3.
55. Allcroft R, Uvarov O. Parenteral administration of copper compounds to cattle with special reference to copper glycine (copper amino-acetate). Vet Rec 1959;71:797–810.

56. Maas J, Peauroi JR, Tonjes T, et al. Intramuscular Selenium Administration in Selenium-Deficient Cattle. J Vet Intern Med 1993;7:342–8.
57. Gonzalez-Rivas PA, Lean GR, Chambers M, et al. A Trace Mineral Injection before Joining and Lambing Increases Marking Percentages and Lamb Weights on Diverse Farms in Victoria, Australia. Animals 2023;13:178.
58. Hall JA, Bobe G, Vorachek WR, et al. Effects of feeding selenium-enriched alfalfa hay on immunity and health of weaned beef calves. Biol Trace Elem Res 2013; 156:96–110.
59. Hall JA, Van Saun RJ, Nichols T, et al. Comparison of selenium status in sheep after short-term exposure to high-selenium-fertilized forage or mineral supplement. Small Rumin Res 2009;82:40–5.
60. Helmer C, Hannemann R, Humann-Ziehank E, et al. A case of concurrent molybdenosis, secondary copper, cobalt and selenium deficiency in a small sheep herd in Northern Germany. Animals 2021;11:1864.

Trace Minerals Nutrition in Goats

David G. Pugh, DVM, MS, MAG, Dipl ACT, ACVIM (Nutrition), ACVM (Parasitology)

KEYWORDS

- Trace minerals • Goat • Trace mineral deficiency • Trace mineral disease

KEY POINTS

- Trace mineral diseases in goats are described in this article.
- The diagnosis and prevention of trace mineral diseases in goats are described in this article.
- The need for feeding trace mineral at adequate dietary concentrations is described in this article.

INTRODUCTION

Trace mineral (TM) deficiency and associated diseases and/or poor production are less commonly encountered in goats than problems associated with diets deficient in energy, protein, or macromineral deficiency. Although many trace minerals have been discovered that are required for goats, the author will confine this discussion to the eight that are of clinical relevance in general veterinary practice.[1–3] These 8 trace minerals are copper (Cu), molybdenum, cobalt (Co), iron (Fe), iodine (I), zinc (Zn), manganese, and selenium (Se). Deficiencies that result in clinical signs occur slowly over time and are rarely associated with the dramatic effects on productivity and body condition, or body condition scores. In some cases of mineral deficiency, collection of peripheral blood or plasma, or a liver biopsy where the collected tissue can be analyzed properly for specific mineral concentrations may be a diagnostic tool, along with dietary evaluation, physical examination, clinical signs, and a complete case history when making a specific diagnosis.[1–4]

COPPER

Cu is required by goats for the growth and production of bone, cartilage, and tendons, for normal hepatic function, for the formation of melanin pigment, for energy metabolism, for transportation/movement of Fe in the body in hemoglobin production, and possibly for the metabolic processes in the body.[2–4]

SouthernTraxx Veterinary Services, PO Box 26, Waverly, AL 36879, USA
E-mail address: dgpugh@southerntraxx.com

Vet Clin Food Anim 39 (2023) 535–543
https://doi.org/10.1016/j.cvfa.2023.05.006
0749-0720/23/© 2023 Elsevier Inc. All rights reserved.

vetfood.theclinics.com

Cu deficiencies can be primary (as a result of low Cu intake) or secondary (resulting by high dietary intakes of molybdenum, sulfur, and Fe, or other substances in feedstuffs).[1,4,5] In the anaerobic conditions of the goat's rumen, Cu, molybdenum, and sulfur form thiomolybdates, which reduce Cu availability to be absorbed and used by the body, which may result in reduced functioning of the enzymes needed for specific biochemical reactions. Clinical signs are the end result of impairment of normal metabolism.[2] Other, less common factors that alter Cu absorption and availability include excess dietary cadmium, Se, Zn, vitamin C, and Zn supplementation in diets (>100 ppm). These dietary "conditions" can also reduce Cu liver. Roughage grown on "improved pastures" (fertilized, limed) is more likely to be deficient. Liming reduces Cu uptake by plants. Many fertilizers contain both molybdenum and sulfur; thus, pasture improvement practices should be carefully evaluated in order to further predispose compromised health. Good-quality lush grass forages may have lowered available Cu than stored forages, such as dry hay, and legumes have more available Cu than most grasses.[1,4,6]

Signs of either "Conditioned" or "Primary" Cu deficiency include microcytic anemia, heart disease and failure, infertility, increased susceptibility to disease, poor or less than optimal productivity (ie, depressed growth, decreased milk production), enlarged joints, lameness, gastric ulcers, diarrhea, lighter hair color, and possibly poor-quality hair in fiber-producing goats.[1,2,6–9] These signs appear to be more severe with primary Cu deficiencies than with "conditioned deficiency" (eg, lowered Cu-molybdenum ratio). Excessive sulfur can elicit several TM deficiencies, including Cu, and thus should always be assessed via complete dietary analysis.

Goats should be offered TM or mineral mixtures free choice, preferably that are designed for goats. When a mineral is designed for sheep (with low to absent added Cu and added molybdenum) as the only dietary for supplemental source minerals, Cu intake may be inadequate for normal goat health. Although Cu is absorbed more efficiently in young animals than in adults, deficiency-associated disease and suboptimal production are usually more common in young, growing animals.[1,4]

Kids born from Cu-deficient does may develop swayback or Enzootic Ataxia. This condition in kids can be diagnosed from birth to 3 months of age. With this condition, kids experience a progressive hindlimb ataxia, with possible ascending paralysis, decreased nursing, muscle atrophy, weakness, and possibly death. Severely affected kids can die within 3 to 4 days of the onset of clinical signs in extreme cases. Necropsy and histologic findings of spinal cord myelin degeneration and cavitations of cerebral white matter are confirmative of this condition. Cu analysis of liver tissue at necropsy in affected neonates will usually be lower than normal and may aid in diagnosis. Prevention and treatment require Cu supplementation (oral supplements, Cu needles, a TM mixture, or injectable Cu) and attainment of a good dietary Cu-to-molybdenum ratio for pregnant goats in areas where this condition is suspected.

In order to determine if Cu deficiency of the diet is the cause of any of this disease, a complete production and dietary history must be attained, a complete and thorough physical examination must be performed, and the entire diet must be evaluated. A dietary evaluation should include a proximate analysis and mineral analysis of all feedstuffs for Cu, molybdenum, and other complicating minerals. Collected samples should be placed into "Ziplock" plastic bags. Where dietary Cu deficiency is suspected, the Cu, molybdenum, sulfur, and Fe concentrations of the diet should be determined from all feeds. Diseases associated with Cu deficiency should be suspected when animals are grazing pasture grass with Cu less than 3 to 5 ppm on a dry matter basis, or where molybdenum is more than 10 ppm on a dry matter basis, and/or sulfur exceeds 2000 ppm, on a dry matter basis.

When attempting to make a definitive diagnosis of Cu deficiency, plasma analysis is a more reliable indicator of body Cu status than is either serum or whole blood. When evaluating blood Cu concentrations of individual goats or multiple members of a herd, the clinician should be reminded that Cu concentrations can be elevated with stress or disease. In cases where serum, plasma Cu concentrations are overtly low and animals are unaffected by stress or sampling, dietary Cu deficiency should be strongly considered. When serum Cu concentrations are found to be within normal values for the laboratory performing the analysis, dietary Cu deficiency would be less likely a cause of clinical signs. However, in cases where whole blood, serum, and/or plasma analysis shows a normal concentration of Cu, yet dietary molybdenum is high or if the Cu-to-molybdenum ratio is less than 4:1, a conditioned Cu deficiency may exist. Dietary Cu-to-molybdenum ratio should be maintained between 5:1 and 10:1. Liver tissue, via biopsy on antemortem goats, or that collected at necropsy, is the best tissue to determine body Cu status. Limitations on the diagnostic value of liver tissue are the reluctance of both clinicians and owners to collect biopsy samples and that liver Cu concentrations are a poor indicator of short-term Cu dietary inadequacies or balance.[1,10] When liver Cu is marginal, but plasma or serum Cu is in the normal range, dietary Cu supplementation should still be recommended, but the herd should be closely monitored in order to not precipitate Cu toxicity. Whenever the clinician suspects a herd problem, samples should be collected both randomly and from those showing clinical signs. Cu deficiency is diagnosed if the blood Cu concentration is less than 0.7 mg/dL or the liver concentration is less than 80 mg/kg dry weight.[5,11]

For optimal production, dietary Cu should range from 4 and 15 ppm. In areas where Cu deficiency is suspected, goats should be offered a mineral mixture with 0.5% Cu sulfate, free choice.[1,4] If additional dietary Cu is required, the clinician should consider the use of orally administered Cu needles, minerals, or supplements containing chelated Cu, or injectable minerals. All forms of Cu supplementation should be used carefully. Cu oxide needles appear to have positive value in the control of internal parasites in goats.[12] Some dwarf breeds of goats may require more dietary Cu than other breeds.[2]

Cu toxicity is relatively rare in goats as compared with sheep. Goats appear to be more "cowlike" in their susceptibility to Cu toxicity than sheep. Signs of Cu toxicity in goats include increased respiration, depression, weakness, hemoglobinuria, icterus, and acute death.[1,2,4] Like in most ruminants, in goats, the dietary and absorbed Cu can accumulate in the liver in proportion to the ratio of Cu to molybdenum in the diet and for the duration of dietary Cu exposure.[2] Cu "dumping" from a saturated liver secondary to episodes of stress or sudden weather changes (eg, cold or heat stress), particularly in the late-pregnant does, or disease causes hemolysis and anemia icterus, kidney failure, liver necrosis, and in severe cases, death of the goat.[2]

ZINC

Zn deficiency is among the more common dietary inadequacies encountered in clinical medicine of goats. Marginal Zn intake, as in other trace minerals, is the most common cause of deficiency. Diets with excessive oxalates, phytates, calcium, cadmium, Fe, molybdenum, and some phosphorus complexes all may reduce Zn availability from the diet and can cause "conditioned" Zn deficiency.[1,9] Conversely, the availability of Zn may be enhanced by diets rich in vitamin C, lactose, and citrate. Zn concentrations are usually higher in legumes than in grasses. Legumes, however, commonly contain large amounts of calcium, which may suppress Zn availability, aiding in a conditioned deficiency. Zn tends to be less available from cereal grain, probably owing to the large amounts of phosphates.

The clinical signs of Zn deficiency include parakeratosis, depressed milk production, impaired appetite, poor feed utilization, slowed growth, increased susceptibility to hoof diseases (ie, foot rot, foot scald), swollen joints, lower than expected reproductive performance, reduced testicular development and size, overgrowth of the dental pad, and alterations in some fat-soluble vitamin requirements and metabolism (ie, vitamin A and E).[1,6,8,9] Cases of Zn-associated parakeratosis may cause reduced growth rate, wrinkled skin, swollen hocks, rough hair coat; hair loss on the head, limbs, and scrotum; and fissures of the feet.[1,2,13,14] Pruritis may or may not be present. The predominant histologic lesions are hyperkeratosis and parakeratosis.[2,11,13,15] Male goats and certain breeds (ie, Pigmy) appear more sensitive to marginal Zn intake and Zn responsive dermatitis.[2]

Whenever Zn deficiency is suspected, the clinician should perform a complete physical examination of all affected animals and the diet and have all dietary components analyzed and evaluated. If Zn deficiency is still suspected, serum or plasma should be collected, handled appropriately, and analyzed for Zn concentrations. Blood drawn for Zn analysis should be collected in a special tube that does not have a butyl rubber stopper. Hemolysis may also alter the ability to accurately interpret Zn status from the collected blood. Liver samples, collected via liver biopsy, is more invasive and carries more risk to the goat, but will usually yield reliable results concerning Zn status. In cases of Zn suspected parakeratosis, a biopsy of the affected area indicating parakeratosis coupled with properly collected serum Zn concentrations of less than 0.8 ppm is diagnostic.[1,2,4]

Diets containing 20 to 50 ppm of Zn are usually sufficient for diets free of calcium or phosphate excesses. Trace mineral-salt mixes with 0.5% to 2% Zn usually prevent deficiency. In these cases where "conditioned" Zn deficiency exists, a chelated form of Zn may be indicated. Removing legumes and cereal grains from the diet and feeding grass, hay, and commercially prepared concentrate feeds (with added Zn) are usually preventative.[11] Treatment may include the daily supplementation of Zn sulfate or Zn methionine daily in the diet for severe cases, or their addition to a salt/mineral mixture offered choice. If calcium makes up 1.5% of the diet, then a form of chelated Zn should be administered or added to a premixed salt supplement. Some response to Zn supplementation should be observed within 14 days, although goats with suspected hereditary malabsorption of Zn may require 1 to 3 months before resolution of most clinical signs.[1,14]

In cases of individual goats with parakeratosis, or for flocks with significant numbers of afflicted animals, adding Zn in the form of zinc sulfate (1 g/d orally) to the diet may be an effective dietary treatment. Zn toxicity is rare under most commonly encountered diets and conditions.[4]

SELENIUM

Se is another of the more common TM deficiencies encountered in routine goat medicine. Dietary Se's absorption from the small intestine is enhanced by adequate dietary levels of vitamins E and A and histidine. Dietary excesses of arsenic, calcium, vitamin C, Cu, nitrates, sulfates, and unsaturated fats appear to depress Se absorption. Legumes are usually better sources of Se than are grasses, which, in turn, are superior sources as compared with cereal grains. Alkaline soils or improved pastures with frequent liming tend to have greater Se uptake by plants, whereas forages grown in areas of high rainfall and acidic soils are usually low or marginal in Se content. Se content of pasture is lowest in the spring and higher in the fall and winter. Irrigation, nitrogen, and phosphorus fertilization may decrease Se uptake and concentration in forages. Early spring, fast-growing forages, particularly in those grown on marginal to Se deficient soils, will more likely be deficient. Hay analysis is crucial in determining dietary Se intake. Forage with less than 0.1 ppm of Se on a dry matter basis is deficient.[1,2,4]

The signs of Se deficiency include nutritional muscular dystrophy (NMD), retained fetal membranes, and less distinct associated health problems, such as poor growth, weak or premature lambs or kids, depressed immune function, mastitis, and post-partum metritis. NMD, also known as white muscle disease, is caused by a deficiency of Se and/or vitamin E. The disease affects both skeletal and cardiac muscle and is more common in young, rapidly growing goats. Focusing on Se's role in this disease, NMD occurs most commonly in kids less than 6 months old, whose dams were fed an Se-deficient diet and has been reported in neonates. Sudden physical exertion or muscular activity in kids with low Se intake or deficient Se body stores will commonly cause clinical signs of NMD in animals unaccustomed to exercise and often triggers episodes of NMD.[1,16] Some byproducts of cell metabolism, such as peroxides, can cause oxidative damage to body cell membranes. Se is a cofactor in some enzyme systems, such as glutathione peroxidase, that help minimize oxidative damage. Se deficiency can result in a reduction of cellular protection against destructive endogenous peroxides. The Se-requiring glutathione peroxidase system is able to convert these destructive chemicals to benign hydroxy fatty acids. Muscles with high-metabolic activity are most susceptible (eg, heart, diaphragm).[16–18]

Goats with Se-associated NMD most commonly present with either cardiac muscle disease or the more common skeletal muscle form. The cardiac muscle form is characterized by acute onset of recumbency, detection of a heart murmur during auscultation, frothy nasal discharge, pulmonary edema, respiratory distress, and death. The history may include collapse after exercise, inability to nurse, and weakness in affected kids.[16–18] A sequalae of aspiration pneumonia owing to glottis dysfunction and dysphagia may be found on a thorough examination of affected goats.[16] Skeletal and cardiac muscle disease may occur concurrently.[18]

As with other diseases, a complete herd history, discussion and evaluation of the diet, a thorough physical examination of signs, and identification of Se-deficient associated signs are required in order to help make an accurate diagnosis. Serum Se concentrations usually reflect dietary intake over the recent 2 to 4 weeks, thus making it difficult to interpret such results, unless overtly lower than expected levels. Whole-blood Se may be of more diagnostic value than serum, as it reflects Se intake over the past 3 to 4 months. In cases of herd Se-associated problems, a collection of 10% of the goat herd should have blood collected for Se analysis. Analysis of red blood cell glutathione peroxidase concentrations is highly correlated with Se concentration and is a useful diagnostic test, if available. If this test is available for use in these cases, the clinician should test for serum Se levels, which may be of value for flock assays if the diet has not been altered for 2 weeks to a few months. Serum Se is of questionable value in assessing goats that have experienced any dietary changes. Evaluating whole-blood Se, collected from suspected goats, yields the most reliable and reproducible results. Se concentration in whole blood reflects the Se level of the diet over the red blood cell's life.[1,16] A necropsy finding of friable muscles contains bilaterally symmetric pale streaks, with regions of degeneration and mineralization. The myocardium may have similar gross lesions. Histologic evaluation of collected muscle samples shows hyaline degeneration, necrosis, and mineralization.[16,17,19] Liver Se concentration is an excellent route to determine adequacy of dietary Se. In cases of suspected NMD, elevated creatine kinase and AST may be elevated in cases of subclinical NMD but is not specific for this condition.[16,17]

Se is readily transferred across the placenta and also is present in colostrum; thus, supplementation of pregnant animals will aid in the reduction of NMD in neonates. Se (and vitamin E) can also be incorporated in mineral mixes that are fed free choice to pregnant and lactating ewes. Diets containing 0.1 to 0.3 ppm of Se are usually adequate for most goats. In areas/regions where Se deficiency has been diagnosed, mineral-salt mixes should contain between 24 and 90 ppm Se, and injectable vitamin E and Se preparations may be given.[1,4] Se toxicity may occur, but deficiency is the more common problem. Toxicity is characterized by anorexia, depression, incoordination, hoof abnormalities, and death.

COBALT

Co toxicity is very rare in goats under practical conditions. Dietary Co is required by goats, as a component of vitamin B12, which is synthesized by rumen bacteria. Available Co is usually in adequate supply in most forages produced in North America but may become deficient in some highly organic and/or poorly drained soils. Inadequate dietary intake of Co is seen as a B12 deficiency rarely encountered in goat medicine. Signs of Co deficiency include inappetence, emaciation, excessive ophthalmic discharge, anemia and pale mucosa, "wasting disease," and, along with phosphorus, Cu deficiencies, and/or chronic parasitism, may be part of the pathogenicity of white liver disease. A diagnosis of Co deficiency may be suggested by finding a diet essentially absent of Co. Necropsy of affected animals may reveal a fatty liver. A confirmative diagnosis can be made based on Co less than 0.06 ppm in the diet, clinical signs, and an increase in serum or urinary methylmalonic acid, and lower than normal serum vitamin B12 and liver Co concentrations. Unfortunately, few veterinary diagnostic laboratories perform all of these tests. A diet with a 0.1 ppm Co level is adequate for most stages of goat production. In the rare event that Co deficiency is diagnosed, a Co-supplemented TM mixture should be fed ad lib.[1]

IRON

Fe is an important component of hemoglobin, and a deficiency can result in microcytic-hypochromic anemia, slowed growth, and poor production in goats. Neonates are born with minimal Fe stores in goats and is quite rare under grazing conditions. Heavily parasitized goats, kids raised in total confinement and fed a milk replacer deficient in Fe, and/or goats deprived of access to pasture and earth-floored stalls or paddocks may become deficient. Treatment for Fe deficiency should include identifying and correcting the primary cause (eg, dietary deficiency, parasitism), possibly using Fe dextran (150 mg intramuscularly at 2- to 3-week intervals).[15] Parenteral Fe dextran may be toxic, and it should be used cautiously when needed.[15] The Fe requirement is generally 30 to 40 ppm of the diet.

IODINE

I deficiency is rare except in geographic regions with sandy soil and where heavy rainfall is encountered.[1,4] Ingestion of calcium in excess, arsenic, fluorine, potassium, rubidium, cyanogenic glycosides, methylthiouracil, nitrates, perchlorates, soybean meal, thiocyanates, and cruciferous plants also may induce I deficiency. Overt signs of I deficiency include goiter, poor growth, depressed milk yield, pregnancy toxemia, abortion, stillbirths, retained placenta, irregular estrus cycles, infertility, depressed libido, birth of small, weak, either hairless or sparsely haired kids, and kids born with enlarged thyroid glands. Affected kids can be treated with 3 to 6 drops of I (Lugol solution) daily for 7 days. As a congenitally enlarged thyroid is also a problem unassociated with dietary I, dietary I must evaluated in order to make an accurate diagnosis. Familial goiter occurs in Dutch goats, and Nubian and Angora goats, and possibly other breeds.[1,4] Goiter also may be caused by congenital defects or ingestion of goitrogens in the diet. A thorough examination of the diet along with serum or plasma thyroxine will aid in determining if dietary I requirements are being met. A diagnosis of I deficiency can be augmented by identifying protein-bound I in serum (normal serum protein-bound I for adult ewes is 2.4–4 µg/dL serum).[4] I levels of 0.8 ppm for lactating animals and 0.2 ppm for nonlactating does in the diet usually meet all needs. Applying I (tincture or Lugol, 1–2 mL) to the skin of a pregnant doe weekly may be useful in I-deficient areas, particularly in small flocks for preventing I deficiency–induced hypothyroidism. I in the form of iodates is absorbed more readily than iodides. I is readily absorbed, so most sources will work well in salt-mineral mixtures or feed supplements. In herds/flocks known to be at risk for marginal to deficient I intake, potassium iodide (150–200 mg) may be administered at 60 and again at 30 days before kidding.[1,4] Providing a good-quality I-containing TM supplement and removing pregnant animals from pastures containing goitrogenous plants decreases the occurrence of goiter. Feeding kelp or related plants have been associated with hyperthyroidism; therefore, such supplementation should be used carefully.[2]

TRACE MINERAL SUPPLEMENTATION

TM salt in block or loose form is composed of NaCl (usually 98% to 99%) with added trace minerals. The nutritionist or clinician should carefully evaluate the type of salt-mineral supplement that is being offered to goats to insure it meets the needs as a supplement for the remainder of the diet for the production status. Goats maintained in dry lots usually consume more than required to meet needs, whereas those that graze or browse on range consume less. Although commonly used, salt blocks are inappropriate for goats, and their use can lead to inadequate mineral intake and the occasional broken tooth.

Complete mineral mixtures in a "loose" nonblock form are preferred for all classes of goats, but will be most beneficial for growing, breeding bucks and does, pregnant, and lactating animals. Intake of a loose mineral mixtures can be predicted by weighing the mineral being offered weekly and dividing by the total animals allowed to consume it. If goats appear to be underconsuming a mineral supplement, the addition of corn, molasses, or soybean meal may enhance uptake. If too much of the mineral mixture is being consumed, adding white salt will usually curtail intake. Mineral supplementation should be based on the individual farms, forage analysis, stage of production, and breed. As a general guide, mineral supplementation should be year-round.[1]

CLINICS CARE POINTS

- The most encountered trace mineral–deficient diseases throughout North America are associated with dietary copper, zinc, and selenium inadequacy.
- Cobalt, iodine, and iron deficiencies are also seen in goats on a regional basis or associated with diseases (ie, iron-internal parasitism).
- Diagnosis of trace mineral deficiency was shown to be made by acquiring a well-discussed history of the problem, complete physical examination, blood collection for a complete

blood count, blood biochemistries, serum/blood collection for trace mineral analysis, possible biopsy for histopathology (ie, zinc, skin), liver biopsy for specific mineral analysis, necropsy (both gross and histologic evaluation), and a complete evaluation of all dietary sources for trace minerals.

DISCLOSURE

The author has nothing to disclose.

REFERENCES

1. Gurung NK, Rush JR, Pugh DG. Chapter 2 - Feeding and Nutrition. In: Pugh DG, N Baird A, Edmondson M, et al, editors. Sheep, goat, and cervid medicine. 3rd edition. Kansas City: Elsevier; 2020. p. P15–44.
2. Pugh DG, Waldridge BM. Goat and llama trace mineral nutrition. Proceed AABP/ AASRP; 2004. p. 112–3.
3. Haenlein GFW, Anke M. Mineral and trace mineral element research in goats: A review. Small Rumin Res 2011;95(1):2–19.
4. Huston JE, White RG, Bequette B, et al. Nutrient Requirements of Small Ruminants: sheep, goats, cervids, and new world camelids. In: Animal nutrition series. NRC of the National Academies; 2007. p. 112–49. Chapter 7.
5. Shen X, Song C, Wu T. Effects of Nano-copper on Antioxidant Function in Copper-Deprived Guizhou Black Goats. Bio Trace Min Res 2021;199:2201–7.
6. Mayasula VK, Arunachalam A, Babatunde SA, et al. Trace minerals for improved performance: a review of Zn and Cu supplementation effects on male reproduction in goats. Trop Anim Health Prod 2021;53:491.
7. Almeida V, Lima TS, Silva-Fiho GB, et al. Copper deficiency in dairy goats and kids. Pesq Vet Bras 2022;42:1–7.
8. Jubril AJ, Kadri ZO, Adekunle LA. A preliminary study on copper and zinc levels and associated haematological changes in the blood of goats slaughtered at Bodija Abattoir, Nigeria. Anim Res Int 2019;16(2):3393–400.
9. Hill GM, Shannon MC. Copper and Zinc Nutritional Issues for Agricultural Animal Production. Biol Trace Element Res 2019;188:148–59.
10. Noorman L, Antonis A, Jorritsma R, et al. Treatment of copper deficiency in Texel-crossbred sheep by the feeding of a concentrate formulated for dairy cows. Vlaams Diergeneeskundig Tijdschrift 2020;89(6):325–8.
11. Baird AN, Shipley CF. Chapter 10 – Diseases of the Integumentary System. In: Pugh DG, N Baird A, Edmondson M, et al, editors. Sheep, goat, and cervid medicine. 3rd edition. Kansas City: Elsevier; 2020. p. 221–50.
12. LA Starkey LA, Pugh DA. Chapter 6 - Gastrointestinal Parasitism. In: Pugh DG, N Baird A, Edmondson M, et al, editors. Sheep, goat, and cervid medicine. 3rd edition. Kansas City: Elsevier; 2020. p. 63–96.
13. Scott DW, Smith MC, Manning TO. Caprine dermatology. Part II. Viral, nutritional, environmental, and congenitohereditary disorders. Comp Cont Ed Pract 1985;6: S473.
14. Krametter-Froetscher R, Hauser S, Baumgartner W. Zinc-responsive dermatosis in goats suggestive of hereditary malabsorption: two field cases. Vet Dermatol 2005;16:269.
15. Bratzlaff K, Henlein G, Huston J. Common nutritional problems feeding the sick goat. In: Naylor JM, Ralston SL, editors. Large animal clinical nutrition. St Louis: Mosby; 1991. p. p351–6.

16. Baird AN, Shipley CF. Chapter 11- Diseases of the Musculoskeletal System. In: Pugh DG, N Baird A, Edmondson M, et al, editors. Sheep, goat, and cervid medicine. 3rd edition. Kansas City: Elsevier; 2020. p. 251–80.
17. Newhard DK, Bayne JE, Passler T. Chapter 17- Diseases of the Cardiovascular System. In: Pugh DG, N Baird A, Edmondson M, et al, editors. Sheep, goat, and cervid medicine. 3rd edition. Kansas City: Elsevier; 2020. p. 439–60.
18. Smart ME, Cymbaluk NF. Trace Minerals. In: Naylor JM, Ralston SL, editors. Large animal clinical nutrition. St Louis: Mosby; 1991. p. 55–67.
19. Edmondson AJ, Norman BB, Suther D. Survey of state veterinarians and state veterinary diagnostic laboratories for selenium deficiency and toxicosis in animals. J Am Vet Med Assoc 1993;202:865.

Common Toxicosis

John P. Buchweitz, PhD, DABT[a,b],*, Rachel Sheffler, DVM[a,b],
Birgit Puschner, DVM, PhD, DABVT[a,b]

KEYWORDS

- Ruminant • Trace mineral • Toxicosis • Bovine • Camelid • Caprine • Ovine

KEY POINTS

- Accurate diagnosis is the key to approaching a potential poisoning case.
- Trace mineral excesses in feed may occur as a result of over- or mis-formulation.
- Soil mineral contaminants may be taken up by plants and animals thus affecting total mineral intake and should be considered when completing ration assessments.
- Trace minerals interact with a broad spectrum of enzymes responsible for a diverse array of cellular and physiologic functions for which adverse impacts could have consequential effects.
- A complex web of mineral-mineral interactions exists, and interpretation of a single mineral result may not provide a complete clinical picture compared to trace mineral panel assessment.

INTRODUCTION

Intoxications in ruminants are infrequent, but when they present, extensive diagnostic, therapeutic, and management measures are required. Accurate diagnosis is the key to approaching a potential poisoning case. Unfortunately, no single procedure will test for all toxicants, and these cases require a multifaceted approach to assemble and solve a diagnostic puzzle. A complete case history, clinical and clinicopathological data, postmortem findings, chemical analyses, and bioassay findings all provide pieces of this puzzle.

Trace mineral toxicoses in ruminants may occur with excess dietary or injectable supplementation, feed mixing errors, through consumption of nutrient-rich or contaminated soil, or grazing plants grown on these aforementioned soils. Excess mineral consumption may result in dietary mineral imbalances through altered absorption and bioavailability of one or more other nutrient minerals. It is well-established that

---

[a] Department of Pathobiology and Diagnostic Investigation, College of Veterinary Medicine, Michigan State University, East Lansing, MI 48824, USA; [b] MSU Veterinary Diagnostic Laboratory, 4125 Beaumont Road, Lansing, MI 48910, USA
* Corresponding author. MSU Veterinary Diagnostic Laboratory, 4125 Beaumont Road, Lansing, MI 48910.
E-mail address: buchwei2@msu.edu

Vet Clin Food Anim 39 (2023) 545–557
https://doi.org/10.1016/j.cvfa.2023.06.006
0749-0720/23/© 2023 Elsevier Inc. All rights reserved.

complex nutrient mineral interactions occur in animal feed and, more specifically, in the forestomach environment. These dietary imbalances impact both short- and long-term animal health and performance.

Toxic residues in food animals may pose a public health risk in edible products, and practitioners may have to navigate publicity, regulatory, and medico-legal issues. Veterinary toxicology laboratories are crucial in advising the practitioner regarding appropriate diagnostic steps and evaluating public health risks.

In this article, we review and organize existing data from trace mineral poisonings in ruminants, identify factors that influence toxicity, describe the clinical signs attributable to various mineral toxicoses, and provide diagnostic threshold criteria for establishing toxicosis.

DISCUSSION
Cobalt

Cobalt is an essential element in the composition of vitamin B_{12} (cobalamins). Ruminants require 0.10 to 0.15 mg/kg diet for the sufficient synthesis of vitamin B_{12} by ruminal microorganisms to meet the animal's dietary needs.[1] However, the recommended maximum tolerable concentration of cobalt in feed based on animal indexes of health is 25 mg/kg dry matter for both cattle and sheep.[1] The maximum safe daily dose of cobalt is reported as 0.88 mg/kg body weight given orally and 3 to 8 mg/kg body weight cobalt chloride injection in calves[2,3]

Toxicoses are rare because of the low concentrations of cobalt normally observed in animal diets.[1] However, suspected cases have been reported in both cattle and sheep and have resulted from errors in formulation or injection.[2,4] Myocardial degeneration has been experimentally induced in guinea pig and rabbit models following cobalt injection and pale myocardium has been reported in sheep; the development of cardiac pathology with cobalt overexposure warrants further investigation in ruminants.[5] Dietary supplementation with methionine or cysteine has been shown to alleviate cobalt toxicosis by chelating cobalt in the rumen and decreasing its absorption.[6,7] Adverse effects associated with cobalt excesses are presented in **Table 1** and diagnostic criteria for establishing toxicosis are presented in **Table 2**.

Copper

Copper metabolism is unique in ruminants because of the delicate interaction between molybdenum, sulfur, and dietary copper that impacts the absorption and bioavailability of these trace nutrients. Copper is an integral part of many important enzymes involved in critical biological processes such as antioxidant activity, formation of connective tissue, iron metabolism, cellular respiration, catecholamine biosynthesis, formation of myelin, melanin pigment and keratin, and maintenance of the immune system.[8,9] Cattle require 15.7 and 10 mg/kg copper dry matter in the diet of lactating dairy and beef cattle respectively to meet the animal's dietary need. Maximum tolerable dietary copper concentrations for cattle are 40 mg/kg diet unless high dietary molybdenum and sulfur concentrations are present.[10] Copper requirements in small ruminants vary by species. Goats require 15 to 25 mg/kg copper dry matter while sheep require 4 to 8 mg/kg copper dry matter. The maximum tolerable dietary limit of copper in goats and sheep respectively is 40 and 15 mg/kg dry matter. These tolerable limits are valid assuming normal dietary concentrations of molybdenum (1–2 mg/kg dry matter) and sulfur (1.5–2.5 g/kg sulfur).[11] Sources of copper that can contribute to overexposure include mineral mixtures in feeds, milk replacer, copper sulfate as an anthelminthic and as a foot bath, pasture fertilizers,

Table 1
Clinical signs of cobalt-related toxicosis

Species	Clinical Signs
Cattle[47–52]	Loss of appetite, loss of body weight, listlessness, and death
Sheep[5,52]	Loss of body weight, death

Table 2
Diagnostic criteria/thresholds for assessing cobalt-related toxicosis

Species	Diet (mg/kg) DM	Blood (μg/mL)	Liver (μg/g) dry	Kidney (μg/g) dry
Cattle[1,2,51]	>25	>0.4	>80	>75
Sheep[2,5]	>25	>0.4	>400	>75

Table 3
Clinical signs of copper-related toxicosis

Species	Clinical Signs
Cattle[52–55]	Anorexia, icterus, dehydration, hemoglobinuria, oliguria, constipation, diarrhea, rumen hypotony
Sheep[16,56–58]	Depression, anorexia, thirst, rumen stasis, weakness, recumbency, hemoglobinuria, icterus, edema around the ears, death within 1–2 d
Goat[59]	Anorexia, recumbency, paddling, vocalization
Camelid[18,60]	Anorexia, recumbency, dullness, regurgitation, grinding of teeth, diarrhea, sunken eyes

Table 4
Diagnostic criteria/thresholds for assessing copper-related toxicosis include the following

Species	Diet (mg/kg) DM	Blood (μg/mL)	Serum (μg/mL)	Liver (μg/g) dry	Kidney (μg/g) dry
Cattle[1,2,19,53,61]	>40		>1.2	>1000	>40
Sheep[1,2,56]	>15	>4.9	>1.2	>900	>100
Goats[2,11,17,59]	>40		>1.2	>500	>40
Camelids[18,60,62]	>40			>650	

Table 5
Clinical signs of iodine-related toxicosis

Species	Clinical Signs
Cattle[22,24,62–64]	Lacrimation, coryza, conjunctivitis, coughing, nasal discharge exophthalmos, hair loss, thyroid enlargement

feeding poultry litter, contamination of soils and vegetation near mining and refining operations, copper oxide boluses, copper wire boluses, and injectable copper supplementation.[12,13]

Acute copper poisoning, which is less frequently reported, is a result of sudden exposure to massive doses of copper, typically after oral or parenteral administration of excessive amounts of soluble copper salts.[8,9,14,15] Chronic copper poisoning is much more common and a result of chronic overexposure and/or insufficient excretion of excess copper.[16] Chronic copper poisoning, including the clinical, clinicopathological, and pathologic changes are well documented; while they result from chronic exposure to copper, onset of clinical signs is sudden with possible death within 1 to 2 days. A stressful event, such as transportation, pregnancy, lactation, handling, disease, or malnutrition, can trigger the breakdown of copper-containing lysosomes resulting in severe hepatocellular disease and subsequent release of copper from the liver. This sudden hepatic copper efflux leads to an acute hemolytic crisis due to oxidative damage and lysis of erythrocytes that results in renal failure that rapidly progresses to sudden death.[12,13]

Chronic copper poisoning is well documented in sheep,[16] which are known to be more susceptible to copper excess due to a decreased ability to eliminate copper through the bile.[14,15] Although there is an abundance of clinical data for sheep, there are relatively few published reports of the disease process in goats. Goats are reportedly less susceptible to copper toxicosis than sheep[16] and may not develop hemolysis.[17] One such report highlights several key aspects of naturally occurring disease and treatment in the goat. The most striking finding was an absence of hemolysis in any clinically affected doe.[17] Camelids appear to be less susceptible to copper poisoning than ruminants and do not develop the classic hemolytic crisis noted in other species.[18]

Diagnosis of chronic copper poisoning is based on clinical signs, clinicopathological changes, post-mortem lesions, and evaluation of copper concentrations in liver, kidney, and serum.[19] It is important to note that blood and serum copper concentrations are poor indicators of hepatic copper loading; there is no correlation between hepatic copper concentrations and serum or blood copper concentrations.[20] Acute hepatic necrosis only develops when the liver stores reach a critical threshold leading to the release of copper from the liver and causing transiently high serum copper concentrations.[21] Adverse effects associated with copper excesses are presented in **Table 3** and diagnostic criteria for establishing toxicosis are presented in **Table 4**.

Iodine

Iodine is an essential element in the composition of the thyroid hormones 3,3′,5-triiodothyronine (T3) and 3,3′,5,5′-tetraiodothyronine (T4). Thyroid hormones regulate cell activity in virtually all tissues and are essential for intermediary metabolism, reproduction, growth and development, hematopoiesis, circulation, neuromuscular function, and thermoregulation.[1] Ruminants require 0.25 to 0.50 mg/kg diet with lactating animals requiring more iodine as approximately 10% of dietary intake may be excreted in milk.[1,22]

The recommended maximum tolerable concentration of iodine in feed based on animal indexes of health is 50 mg/kg dry matter for both cattle and sheep.[1] Iodine is a cumulative, chronic poison and the reported tolerable doses are for all sources (feed, dips, supplements, and water).[23] In addition to feed sources, toxicoses have been reported to result from the misuse of ethylenediamine dihydroiodide (EDDI) or potassium iodide for the oral treatment of foot rot, woody tongue (*Actinobacillus lignieresii* infection) and lumpy jaw (*Actinomyces bovis* infection).[24] Paradoxically, exposure to excess iodine (iodism) results in hypothyroidism because of feedback inhibition of T3 synthesis and may result in thyroid gland enlargement.[23,25] For this reason, it is critical to differentiate iodine toxicosis from deficiency in animals exhibiting goiter. Clinical signs and diagnostic criteria for iodism are presented in **Table 5** and **Table 6**, respectively.

Iron

Iron is found to be present in all cells of the body with its major role in both hemoglobin and myoglobin.[1] For each of these biomolecules, either between tissues (hemoglobin) or within tissues (myoglobin), oxygen transport is central.[26] Iron is also found in milk (lactoferrin), the plasma (transferrin), and liver (ferritin and hemosiderin).[23,26] Iron requirements in cattle of all stages is 50 mg/kg bodyweight.[10,27]

The recommended maximum tolerable concentration of iron in feed based on animal indexes of health is 1000 mg/kg for cattle[1,10,27] and 500 mg/kg for sheep.[1] If maintained, these concentrations may lead to long-term liver injury, especially if vitamin E concentrations are low or there are endogenous stores of excess iron.[10,27] High concentrations of iron may also induce secondary deficiencies of cobalt, copper, manganese, selenium or zinc.[2] Clinical signs of iron toxicosis and diagnostic criteria are provided in **Tables 7** and **8**.

Manganese

Manganese is widely distributed in mammalian tissues at very low concentrations and is necessary for the normal development of bone and reproductive processes in both sexes. Manganese is incorporated into several metalloenzymes including pyruvate carboxylase (gluconeogenesis and lipogenesis), superoxide dismutase (oxidative stress), and glycosyltransferase (synthesis of mucopolysaccharides and prothrombin).[23] Beef and dairy cattle require 20 and 40 mg/kg diet, respectively.[10,27] The recommended maximum tolerable concentration of manganese in feed based on animal indexes of health is 2000 mg/kg dry matter feed for both cattle and sheep.[1] There are no studies to date reporting acute toxic effects of manganese in mammals. Chronic exposure may lead to changes listed in **Table 9**. Diagnostic criteria are provided in **Table 10**.

Molybdenum

Molybdenum is an essential component of a group of enzymes known as molybdenum oxotransferases that serve as catalysts for several metabolic oxidation-reduction reactions.[28] The daily intake of molybdenum from the air and drinking water is negligible compared to the absorption of molybdenum from the diet, except in molybdenum mining areas that may have increased environmental molybdenum contamination.[29] Animal feed sources are mostly low in molybdenum, except for marine products and milk from animals grazing on molybdenum-rich pastures.[1,23]

The recommended maximum tolerable concentration of molybdenum in feed based on animal indexes of health is 5 mg/kg dry matter for both cattle and sheep.[1] This maximum concentration varies with species, dietary copper-to-molybdenum ratio, copper status of the animal and dietary concentration of sulfur.[23] The ideal copper-to-molybdenum ratio by concentration in feed is 6:1 with values < 2:1 being toxic.[2] The sulphate-to-molybdenum ratio by concentration should be 100:1.[2] This three-way interaction between copper, molybdenum, and sulfur leads to the formation of a copper thiomolybdate complex in the rumen, thus determining the tolerance to excess molybdenum.[23] Accordingly, molybdenum-containing drugs (eg, ammonium

Table 6
Diagnostic criteria/thresholds for assessing iodine-related toxicosis

Species	Diet (mg/kg) DM	Serum (μg/dL)	Thyroid (μg/g)	Milk (mg/L)
Cattle(acute)[2]	>400	>1000	>5000	
Cattle(chronic)[1,2]	>50	>100	>5000	>1.13
Sheep[1,2]	>50	>4000		>15
Goat[2]		>1200		>35

Table 7
Clinical signs of iron-related toxicosis

Species	Clinical Signs
Cattle[65]	Weight loss, diarrhea, hepatic failure

Table 8
Diagnostic criteria/thresholds for assessing iron-related toxicosis

Species	Diet (mg/kg) DM	Serum (μg/dL)	Liver (μg/g) dry	Kidney (μg/g) dry
Cattle[1,2]	>500	>1800	>2000	>250
Sheep[1,2]	>500			

Table 9
Clinical signs of manganese-related toxicosis

Species	Clinical Signs
Cattle[66,67]	Reduced appetite and growth, anemia, abdominal discomfort
Sheep[2]	Reduced feed intake and growth, reduced hemoglobin formation and iron status in lambs

Table 10
Diagnostic criteria/thresholds for assessing manganese-related toxicosis

Species	Diet (mg/kg) DM	Serum (μg/mL)	Liver (μg/g) dry	Kidney (μg/g) dry
Cattle[1,2]	>2000	>0.08		
Sheep[2,11]	>3000	>3.0	>12.5	>12.5

Table 11
Clinical signs of molybdenum-related toxicosis

Species	Clinical Signs
Cattle[68]	Diarrhea, reduced growth, anemia, stiff gaited lameness, decreased hair pigmentation
Sheep[2]	Diarrhea, steely wool, reduced growth, anemia

tetrathiomolybdate) can be utilized as a therapeutic agent in the treatment of copper accumulation disorders.[30]

In ruminants, excess dietary molybdenum interferes with copper uptake and plasma protein binding. For non-ruminants, additional dietary sulfur may offer protection against excessive dietary molybdenum. However, in ruminants excess sulfur can exacerbate the impairment of copper metabolism.[31] Thus, molybdenum has relatively low toxicity, and molybdenosis (teart) is a disease of secondary copper deficiency due to the molybdenum-copper interactions.[29] Sheep are especially susceptible to molybdenosis because of their lower tolerance of copper and decreased dietary intakes. Serum is considered a useful diagnostic tool to assess molybendosis; however, evidence of copper deficiency is not apparent in serum until severe hepatic copper depletion has occurred. Clinical signs and diagnostic criteria for molybdenum toxicosis are presented in **Table 11** and **Table 12**, respectively.

Selenium

Selenium is essential for the normal function of most organ systems through antioxidant activity, immune modulation, endocrine function, bone metabolism, iodine metabolism, and reproductive processes.[32] Selenium-dependent enzyme systems and selenium binding proteins, such as the glutathione peroxidase, catalyze the reduction of hydrogen peroxide and several organic hydroperoxides by the oxidation of reduced glutathione to oxidized glutathione. This pathway highlights the importance of selenium in the antioxidant defense mechanism. Additionally, selenium is an essential component of normal immune and cardiovascular system function and plays a role in the prevention of some types of cancer.[33,34] Plants are the main source of dietary selenium and vary considerably in their physiologic response to soil selenium concentrations; some plant species are selenium tolerant and accumulate very high concentrations of selenium, but most species are non-accumulators.[35] The maximum concentration of selenium that can be legally added to the diet is reported as 0.3 mg/kg dry matter for ruminants in the United States.[36] The maximum tolerable limit of selenium in the diet of ruminants is 5 mg/kg dry matter.[1]

The Kesterson Reservoir controversy in the 1980s made scientists, regulators, politicians, and the public acutely aware of the importance of selenium as an environmental contaminant.[37] In livestock, acute selenium toxicosis is a result of ingestion of seleniferous accumulator plants or due to excess supplementation by parenteral or oral route.[38,39] Chronic selenosis, also known as alkali disease, occurs after the consumption of diets containing 5 to 40 mg Se/kg over a period of several weeks or months.[40] The relatively wide range between optimal and toxic levels of dietary selenium is based on the varying bioavailabilities of different chemical forms of selenium. Organic selenium accumulates to a greater extent in organs and tissues than inorganic sodium selenite.[39,41] Clinical signs and diagnostic criteria for selenium toxicosis are presented in **Tables 13** and **14**, respectively.

Zinc

Zinc is essential for a wide variety of cellular processes in all cells including the structural and catalytic function of hundreds of enzymes that regulate the major metabolic pathways of the body.[42] It plays a crucial role in cell differentiation, cell division, cell growth, cellular transport, endocrine and immune function, transcription, protein synthesis, RNA and DNA synthesis, DNA replication, and is a cofactor for more than 1000 enzymatic reactions and more than 2000 transcription factors.[42] Dietary zinc requirements in dairy cattle vary by production class ranging from 30 to 63 mg/kg dry matter, while beef cattle and sheep require 30 mg/kg diet for all production

Table 12
Diagnostic criteria/thresholds for assessing molybdenum-related toxicosis

Species	Diet (mg/kg) DM	Serum (µg/mL)	Liver (µg/g) dry	Kidney (µg/g) dry
Cattle[1,2]	>5	>0.1	>5.5	>3
Sheep[1,2]	>5	>2.3	>5.5	>3

Table 13
Clinical signs of selenium-related toxicosis

Species	Clinical Signs
Cattle and sheep[38,39,69–71]	Acute: Depression, dyspnea, labored breathing, abnormal movement and posture, diarrhea, death possible in few hours
Cattle[70,72]	Chronic: Lameness, swelling of coronary bands, hoof deformities, rough hair, loss of hair, inappetence, weight loss, diarrhea, infertility (direct or indirect)

Table 14
Diagnostic criteria/thresholds for assessing selenium-related toxicosis

Species	Diet (mg/kg) DM	Blood (ng/mL)	Serum (µg/mL)	Liver (µg/g) dry	Kidney (µg/g) dry	Hair (µg/g) dry
Cattle[2,69,73]	>10	1.0	0.5	15.5	7.5	1.4
Sheep[1,38,74,75]	>5	1.0	0.8	12.5	7.5	45

Table 15
Clinical signs of zinc-related toxicosis

Species	Clinical Signs
Cattle[76]	Diarrhea, anorexia, pica, polyuria, polydipsia, pneumonia, cardiac arrythmias, and seizures

Table 16
Diagnostic criteria/thresholds for assessing zinc-related toxicosis

Species	Diet (mg/kg) DM	Serum (µg/mL)	Liver (µg/g) dry	Kidney (µg/g) dry
Cattle[1,2,43,61]	>500	>0.1	>500	>250
Sheep[1,2]	>300	>2.3	>30	>200
Goat[11]	>1000			

classes.[10,11] The maximal tolerable zinc concentration is suggested to be 300 mg/kg in sheep and goats and between 300 and 1000 mg/kg diet in cattle.[1] However, zinc antagonism from other minerals and organic compounds in the diet may alter dietary requirements on a herd-by-herd basis.

Zinc poisoning has been reported in cattle and is usually a result of accidental over-supplementation.[43] Excessive concentrations of injectable zinc and zinc-iron boluses, and the addition of zinc to drinking water, salt-mineral blocks, dietary rations, and milk replacer have been associated with zinc toxicosis in cattle.[43–45] Calves are more susceptible to zinc poisoning than adult cattle.

The diagnosis of the early stages of zinc deficiency or toxicosis can be difficult. Zinc concentrations in serum and plasma are the most widely used indicators of zinc status, but they lack repeatability and sensitivity as a diagnostic criterion due to individual animal variability.[46] It is important to note that vacutainer collection tubes with rubber stoppers may artificially increase zinc concentrations in serum and plasma samples as zinc may leach from the rubber. Clinical signs and diagnostic criteria for zinc toxicosis are presented in **Tables 15** and **16**, respectively.

SUMMARY

Toxicoses of trace minerals may occur in ruminant livestock following excessive oral or injectable supplementation, ration formulation errors, or with environmental contamination in nutrient-dense soils and plant material. With many potential etiologies, it is essential to evaluate dietary, environmental, management, and individual animal factors that may contribute to the development of toxicosis. Excessive mineral consumption and dietary imbalances can be detrimental to both short and long-term health and performance which may result in significant economic losses to producers through decreased efficiency of feed conversion, condemnation of carcasses, or death. For these reasons, mineral toxicoses merit continued clinical attention.

CLINICS CARE POINTS

- Trace mineral intoxications in ruminants are relatively infrequent, but can result in acute, and often lethal presentations or chronic illness.

- Intoxications should be suspected if there are multiple animals are affected, or there are unusual clinical signs, or unexplained deaths.

- Chronic trace mineral poisonings are difficult to diagnose because excess exposure may have occurred over a period of weeks to months before clinical signs become noticeable.

- Trace mineral poisonings in ruminants are often complicated and may involve regulatory agencies due to reporting requirements.

- Prompt consultation with a veterinary toxicology laboratory and state veterinary offices can provide significant guidance with respect to establishing a diagnosis and management protocol.

- Mineral toxicoses may present similarly to deficiencies, ie, iodine, therefore it is important to differentiate the conditions with appropriate diagnostic data.

- Evaluation of management protocols, diet, and environment together is key in assessing mineral toxicoses.

DISCLOSURE

The authors have nothing to disclose.

REFERENCES

1. National Research Council. 2005. Mineral Tolerance of Animals: Second Revised Edition, 2005, The National Academies Press; Washington, DC, doi:10.17226/11309.
2. Puls R. Mineral levels in animal health. Diagnostic data. British Columbia (Canada): Sherpa International; 1994.
3. Ely RE, Dunn KM, Huffman CF. Cobalt toxicity in calves resulting from high oral administration. J Anim Sci 1948;7:239–46.
4. Herdt TH, Hoff B. The use of blood analysis to evaluate trace mineral status in ruminant livestock. Veterinary Clinics: Food Animal Practice 2011;27(2):255–83.
5. Andrews ED. Cobalt poisoning in sheep. N Z Vet J 1965;13(4):101–3.
6. Baker DH, Czarnecki-Maulden GL. Pharmacologic role of cysteine in ameliorating or exacerbating mineral toxicities. J Nutr 1987;117(6):1003–10.
7. Southern LL, Baker DH. The effect of methionine or cysteine on cobalt toxicity in the chick. Poult Sci 1981;60(6):1303–8.
8. Gaetke LM, Chow-Johnson HS, Chow CK. Copper: toxicological relevance and mechanisms. Arch Toxicol 2014;88:1929–38. https://doi.org/10.1007/s00204-014-1355-y.
9. Gaetke LM, Chow CK. Copper toxicity, oxidative stress, and antioxidant nutrients. Toxicology 2003;189(1–2):147–63. https://doi.org/10.1016/S0300-483X(03)00159-8.
10. National Research Council. Nutrient Requirements of Dairy Cattle. Seventh Revised Edition. Washington, DC,: The National Academies Press; 2001. https://doi.org/10.17226/9825.
11. National Research Council. Nutrient Requirements of Small Ruminants: Sheep, Goats, Cervids, and New World Camelids. Washington, DC,: The National Academies Press; 2007. https://doi.org/10.17226/11654.
12. Puschner B, Thurmond MC, Choi YKK. Influence of age and production type on liver copper concentrations in calves. J Vet Diagn Invest 2004;16(5):382–7.
13. Robinson FR, Sullivan JM, Brelage DR, et al. Comparison of hepatic lesions in veal calves with concentrations of copper, iron and zinc in liver and kidney. Vet Hum Toxicol 1999;41(3):171–4.
14. Søli NE, Nafstad I, Søli NE, et al. Effects of daily oral administration of copper to goats. Acta Vet Scand 1978;19(4):561.
15. Haywood S, Simpson DM, Ross G, et al. The greater susceptibility of North Ronaldsay sheep compared with Cambridge sheep to copper-induced oxidative stress, mitochondrial damage and hepatic stellate cell activation. J Comp Pathol 2005;133(2–3):114–27.
16. Soli NE, Søli NE. Chronic copper poisoning in sheep. A review of the literature. Nord Vet Med 1980;32(2):75–89.
17. Cornish J, Angelos J, Puschner B, et al. Copper toxicosis in a dairy goat herd. J Am Vet Med Assoc 2007;231(4):586–9.
18. Carmalt JL, Baptiste KE, Blakley B. Suspect copper toxicity in an alpaca. Can Vet J 2001;42(7):554.
19. Bidewell CA, Drew JR, Payne JH, et al. Case study of copper poisoning in a British dairy herd. Vet Rec Case Rep 2013;1(1):e100267.

20. Blakley BR, Hamilton DL. Ceruloplasmin as an indicator of copper status in cattle and sheep. Can J Comp Med 1985;49(4):405.

21. Auza NJ, Olson WG, Murphy MJ, et al. Diagnosis and treatment of copper toxicosis in ruminants. J Am Vet Med Assoc 1999;214(11):1624–8.

22. Miller JK, Swanson EW, Spalding GE. Iodine absorption, excretion, recycling, and tissue distribution in the dairy cow. J Dairy Sci 1975;58(10):1578–93.

23. Suttle NF. Mineral Nutrition of Livestock. 4th Edition. Cambridge,: CABI; 2010. doi: 10.1079/9781845934729.0000.

24. Hillman D, Curtis AR. Chronic iodine toxicity in dairy cattle: Blood chemistry, leukocytes, and milk iodide. J Dairy Sci 1980;63(1):55–63.

25. Newton GL, Barrick ER, Harvey RW, et al. Iodine toxicity. Physiological effects of elevated dietary iodine on calves. J Anim Sci 1974;38(2):449–55.

26. Underwood EJ. Trace Elements in Human and Animal Nutrition. 4th Edition. New York: Academic Press; 2012.

27. National Research Council. Nutrient Requirements of Beef Cattle: Seventh Revised Edition. Washington, DC,: The National Academies Press; 2000. https://doi.org/10.17226/9791.

28. Johnson MK, Garton SD, Oku H. Resonance Raman as a direct probe for the catalytic mechanism of molybdenum oxotransferases. J Biol Inorg Chem 1997;2: 797–803.

29. Barceloux DG, Barceloux DrD. Molybdenum. J Toxicol Clin Toxicol 1999;37(2): 231–7.

30. Gooneratne SR, Howell JM, Gawthorne JM. Intravenous administration of thiomolybdate for the prevention and treatment of chronic copper poisoning in sheep. Br J Nutr 1981;46(3). https://doi.org/10.1079/bjn19810054.

31. Grace ND, Suttle NF. Some effects of sulphur intake on molybdenum metabolism in sheep. Br J Nutr 1979;41(1):125–36.

32. Pecoraro BM, Leal DF, Frias-De-Diego A, et al. The health benefits of selenium in food animals: a review. J Anim Sci Biotechnol 2022;13(1):1–11. https://doi.org/10. 1186/S40104-022-00706-2.

33. Fairweather-Tait SJ, Filippini T, Vinceti M. Selenium status and immunity. Proc Nutr Soc. 2023;82(1):32–8. https://doi.org/10.1017/S0029665122002658.

34. Hosnedlova B, Kepinska M, Skalickova S, et al. A Summary of New Findings on the Biological Effects of Selenium in Selected Animal Species—A Critical Review. Int J Mol Sci 2017;18(10):2209.

35. Terry N, Zayed AM, De Souza MP, et al. Selenium in higher plants. Annu Rev Plant Physiol Plant Mol Biol 2000;51:401–32. https://doi.org/10.1146/annurev.arplant. 51.1.401.

36. Mehdi Y, Dufrasne I. Selenium in Cattle: A Review. Molecules 2016;21(4):545.

37. Ohlendorf HM. The birds of Kesterson Reservoir: a historical perspective. Aquat Toxicol 2002;57(1–2):1–10.

38. Blodgett DJ, Bevill RF. Acute selenium toxicosis in sheep. Vet Hum Toxicol 1987; 29(3):233–6.

39. Tiwary AK, Panter KE, Stegelmeier BL, et al. Naturally occurring acute selenium toxicosis in sheep, International Symposium on Poisonous Plants. In: Poisonous plants : global research and solutions. Wallingford, Oxfordshire, UK; Cambridge, MA: CABI Pub; 2007. http://www.loc.gov/catdir/toc/ecip079/2007003872.html.

40. Olson OE. Selenium toxicity in animals with emphasis on man. J Am Coll Toxicol 1986;5(1):45–70.

41. Shini S, Sultan A, Bryden WL. Selenium Biochemistry and Bioavailability: Implications for Animal Agriculture. Agriculture 2015;5(4):1277–88. https://doi.org/10.3390/AGRICULTURE5041277.

42. Chasapis CT, Spiliopoulou CA, Loutsidou AC, et al. Zinc and human health: An update. Arch Toxicol 2012;86(4):521–34. https://doi.org/10.1007/S00204-011-0775-1/METRICS.

43. Graham TW, Keen CL, Holmberg CA, et al. An Episode of Zinc Toxicosis in Milk-Fed Holstein Bull Calves: Pathologic and Toxicologic Considerations. In: Hurley LS, Keen CL, Lönnerdal B, Rucker RB, editors. Trace Elements in Man and Animals 6. Boston, MA: Springer; 1988. https://doi.org/10.1007/978-1-4613-0723-5_257.

44. Allen JG, Masters HG, Peet RL, et al. Zinc toxicity in ruminants. J Comp Pathol 1983;93(3):363–77. https://doi.org/10.1016/0021-9975(83)90024-5.

45. Jenkins KJ, Hidiroglou M. Tolerance of the Preruminant Calf for Excess Manganese or Zinc in Milk Replacer. J Dairy Sci 1991;74(3):1047–53. https://doi.org/10.3168/JDS.S0022-0302(91)78254-4.

46. Corrigall W, Dalgarno AC, Ewen LA, et al. Modulation of plasma copper and zinc concentrations by disease states in ruminants. Vet Rec 1976;99(20):396–7.

47. Askew HO, Josland SW. The rate of excretion of cobalt by sheep after drenching with cobalt chloride. N Z J Sci Technol Sect A 1937;18:888–92.

48. Becker DE, Smith SE. The level of cobalt tolerance in yearling sheep. J Anim Sci 1951;10(1):266–71.

49. Corrier DE, Rowe LD, Clark DE, et al. Tolerance and effect of chronic dietary cobalt on sheep. Vet Hum Toxicol 1986;28(3):216–9.

50. Keener HA, Percival GP, Mobbow KS, et al. Cobalt tolerance in young dairy cattle. J Dairy Sci 1949;32:527–33.

51. MacLaren APC, Johnston WG, Voss RC. Cobalt poisoning in cattle. Vet Rec 1964; 76:1148–9.

52. Radostits OM, Gay CC, Hinchcliff KW, et al. In: Abutarbush SM, editor. Veterinary medicine: a textbook of the diseases of cattle, horses, sheep, pigs, and goats. 10th edition. Saunders Elsevier; 2007.

53. Gummow B. Experimentally induced chronic copper toxicity in cattle. Onderstepoort J Vet Res 1996;63(4):277–88.

54. Minervino AHH, Barrêto Júnior RA, Ferreira RNF, et al. Clinical observations of cattle and buffalos with experimentally induced chronic copper poisoning. Res Vet Sci 2009;87(3):473–8. https://doi.org/10.1016/J.RVSC.2009.05.002.

55. Tokarnia CH, Döbereiner J, Peixoto PV, et al. Outbreak of copper poisoning in cattle fed poultry litter. Vet Hum Toxicol 2000;42(2):92–5.

56. Arora RG, Andersson L, Bucht RS, et al. Chronic copper toxicosis in sheep, Nord Vet Med, 1977;29(4–5):181-187.

57. Christodoulopoulos G, Roubies N. Diagnosis and treatment of copper poisoning caused by accidental feeding on poultry litter in a sheep flock. Aust Vet J 2007; 85(11):451–3. https://doi.org/10.1111/j.1751-0813.2007.00186.x.

58. Thompson LJ. Copper, In: Gupta RC (ed), Veterinary toxicology: basic and clinical principles, 3rd edition, 2018, 604-608, doi:10.1016/B978-0-12-811410-0.00026-X.

59. Bozynski CC, Evans TJ, Dae YK, et al. Copper toxicosis with hemolysis and hemoglobinuric nephrosis in three adult Boer goats. J Vet Diagn Invest 2009;21(3): 395–400.

60. Abu Damir H, Eldirdiri NI, Adam SEI, et al. Experimental copper poisoning in the camel (Camelus dromedarius). J Comp Pathol 1993;108(2):191–208. https://doi.org/10.1016/S0021-9975(08)80221-6.
61. Counotte G, Holzhauer M, Carp-van Dijken S, et al. Levels of trace elements and potential toxic elements in bovine livers: A trend analysis from 2007 to 2018. PLoS One 2019;14(4):e0214584.
62. Freer M. Nutrient requirements of domesticated ruminants. CSIRO publishing; 2007.
63. Underwood EJ. Trace elements in human and animal nutrition. 4th edition. New York: Academic Press; 1977.
64. Haggard DL, Stowe HD, Conner GH t, et al. Immunologic effects of experimental iodine toxicosis in young cattle. Am J Vet Res 1980;41(4):539–43.
65. House JK, Smith BP, Maas J, et al. Hemochromatosis in Salers Cattle, J Vet Intern Med, 8(2):1994, 105-111, doi:10.1111/j.1939-1676.1994.tb03206.x.
66. Cunningham GN, Wise MB, Barrick ER. Effect of High Dietary Levels of Manganese on the Performance and Blood Constituents of Calves, J Anim Sci, 1966;25(2):532-538, doi:10.2527/jas1966.252532x.
67. Hartman RH, Matrone G, Wise GH. Effect of high dietary manganese on hemoglobin formation. J Nutr 1955;57(3):429–39. https://doi.org/10.1093/jn/57.3.429.
68. Britton JW, Goss H, Chronic molybdenum poisoning in cattle, J Am Vet Med Assoc, 1946;108:176-178.
69. MacDonald DW, Christian RG, Strausz KI, et al. Acute selenium toxicity in neonatal calves. Can Vet J 1981;22(9):279.
70. Raisbeck MF. Selenosis in Ruminants. Vet Clin North Am Food Anim Pract 2020; 36(3):775–89. https://doi.org/10.1016/J.CVFA.2020.08.013.
71. Smith BI, Donovan GA, Rae DO. Selenium toxicosis in a flock of Katahdin hair sheep. Can Vet J 1999;40(3):192.
72. Hosseinion H, Bazargani TT, Nahani J, et al. Selenium poisoning in a mixed flock of sheep and goats in Iran. Trop Anim Health Prod 1972;4(3):173–4. https://doi.org/10.1007/BF02359768/METRICS.
73. Davis TZ, Stegelmeier BL, Panter KE, et al. Toxicokinetics and pathology of plant-associated acute selenium toxicosis in steers. J Vet Diagn Invest 2012;24(2): 319–27. https://doi.org/10.1177/1040638711435407.
74. Davis PA, McDowell LR, Wilkinson NS, et al. Comparative effects of various dietary levels of Se as sodium selenite or Se yeast on blood, wool, and tissue Se concentrations of wether sheep. Small Rumin Res 2008;74(1–3):149–58. https://doi.org/10.1016/J.SMALLRUMRES.2007.05.003.
75. Fessler AJ, Moller G, Talcott PA, et al. Selenium toxicity in sheep grazing reclaimed phosphate mining sites. Vet Hum Toxicol 2003;45(6):294–8.
76. Graham TW, Thurmond MC, Clegg MS, et al. An epidemiologic study of mortality in veal calves subsequent to an episode of zinc toxicosis on a California veal calf operation using zinc sulfate-supplemented milk replacer. J Am Vet Med Assoc 1987;190(10):1296–301.

Moving?

Make sure your subscription moves with you!

To notify us of your new address, find your **Clinics Account Number** (located on your mailing label above your name), and contact customer service at:

Email: journalscustomerservice-usa@elsevier.com

800-654-2452 (subscribers in the U.S. & Canada)
314-447-8871 (subscribers outside of the U.S. & Canada)

Fax number: 314-447-8029

Elsevier Health Sciences Division
Subscription Customer Service
3251 Riverport Lane
Maryland Heights, MO 63043

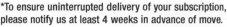

*To ensure uninterrupted delivery of your subscription, please notify us at least 4 weeks in advance of move.

Printed and bound by CPI Group (UK) Ltd, Croydon, CR0 4YY

03/10/2024

01040469-0018